C000216587

AIDS:
THE HOMŒOPATHIC
CHALLENGE

Jonathan Stallick   MHMA

RIBBLE PRESS

Settle, North Yorkshire

1996

ISBN 0 9528531 0 8

Cover illustration by: Ellen Walton

Printed by: Lamberts Printers, Settle, North Yorkshire

Contents

Acknowledgements	viii
Dedication	ix
Preface	x
Foreword	xii
Introduction	1
In At The Deep End	4
Taking The Case	8
Prescribing And Case Management	10
The Layers Model	15
Aetiologies	24
Constitutional Prescribing	24
Drainage	25
Flower Essences	26
Auto-isopathy and Sarcodes	27
Nosodes	27
The Nature Of The Work	32
Psychological Issues	38
The Healing Power Within	43
What Causes Immunodeficiency?	46
Candidiasis	48
Materia Medica	54
A Medical Overview Of Aids	92
Medical Tests And Drugs	99
In Conclusion	108
Bibliography	109
Addresses	111
Remedy Index	113
General Index	115

Agnus Castus   54

Aids Nosode   55

Ambra Grisea   59

Anthracinum   59

Arsenicum Album   60

AZT   60

Calcium Salts   61

Calcarea Carbonica   61

Calc Bromatum   62

Calcarea Arsenicosum   65

Calcarea Phosphorica   66

Calcarea Sulphurica   66

Carbo Vegetabilis   67

Carcinosin   67

China   68

Cocculus   69

Coffea   69

Cyclosporin   70

Echinacea   70

Hydrastis   71

Kali Carbonica   72

Lecithin   72

Leprominium   72

Lycopodium   73

Contents

Medorrhinum	73
Mercurius Corrosivus	74
Mercurius Solubilis	75
Muriatic Acid	76
Natrum Sulphuricum	76
Nitricum Acidum	77
Phosphorus	78
Radium Bromide	81
Rhus Toxicodendron	81
Stannum	82
SVA	83
Syphilinum	83
Thuja	84
Thymus Gland	84
Tuberculinum	87
Typhoidinum	88
Vanadium Metallicum	89
X-Ray	91

My thanks to...

Julie Williams for editing and providing unstinting support throughout; Martin Miles, Deirdre Holmes, Marc Blausten, Shereen Joshua, Misha Norland and Alan Jones for sharing much valuable information; Charles Wansbrough and *Prometheus Unbound*; Anne Organ for her constant encouragement; my parents for being my parents; Peter McDonnell for giving me all kinds of clues as to where my path lies; Lisa Monck, who sadly died in 1994, for providing the initial inspiration for me to break out of a purely 'classical' mould; Kenneth Metson for cheering me on and providing the preface; Richard Kenchington of Ribble Press for taking this project on and getting the draft into shape and ready for the printers.

Dedicated To Lisa Monck

I first met Lisa Monck when I was studying at the College of Homœopathy in London in 1984. She was a bird-like creature, very slim, with fair hair and Scandinavian features and she looked much younger than she was. She was one of the brightest students in our year and we struck up a friendship. After leaving college we lost contact for a while but after a couple of years we met again and I remember Lisa being very excited, if a little coy, about her new way of working with patients.

At college we were taught, basically, a 'classical' approach to homœopathic prescribing i.e. one remedy at a time and wait. So when she described how she was working I could understand her initial shyness. She told me that she had tried the classical approach; she would repertorise faithfully to find the indicated remedy but would be disappointed when she did not get the results she had been led to expect. So, in certain cases, she abandoned this method and experimented with identifying layers, blocks and organ weaknesses and she would then prescribe on several or all of these at once, high potency after high potency of different remedies prescribed consecutively.

At first I was shocked, but when I looked closely at her results I was truly amazed, for she was helping people back to health quickly and efficiently in a way, to my eyes, that was closer to the true spirit of Hahnemann than some of the rigid dogma that has been attributed to him.

Her thinking behind prescriptions was sometimes on the wild side but she was doing what worked. And, I reasoned, what could work for her could also work for me!

It has sometimes seemed to me that homœopaths are quick to criticise the medical profession for narrow mindedness and rigid thinking but are unwilling to look at the same negative aspects in their own back yard. Her original thinking continues to influence many homœopaths.

Thank you Lisa!

Dr Kenneth Metson PhD
Fellow of The Homœopathic Medical Association

Homœopathy is probably the most complete system of alternative medicine ever presented to Man, due to its holistic approach, its philosophy and its huge armamentarium of remedies. By using potentised medicine it becomes dynamic to illness via the vital force and is capable of restoring health by gentle means.

Before we can understand the sufferings of humanity we have to understand ourselves. Not an easy task, but I believe Jonathan has achieved just that, so it makes his dynamis even more so. This man has the courage of his convictions and is now prepared to share his experiences with you.

Some practitioners in our profession may be aghast when reading this text as to the potencies used, the frequency of repetition etc., but I can assure you that when presented with gross pathology you have to make your prescription equal in force. Hence the law of similars (Similia Similibus Curentur) will always persist whatever the sphere.

I have been in practice for some thirty-eight years and have used these methods of prescribing with the greatest results, so I can give my hearty support to Jonathan in his method of prescribing. Jonathan did some of his training under my direction and I feel proud to read this treatise and write this preface.

When one begins their training to become a homœopath we have to rely on our preceptors, books from the masters, and repertorisation. This will only form the basis of the science of homœopathy, so when we eventually enter into practice we then begin to learn the art of homœopathic medicine.

Repertorisation will never supersede the intimate
knowledge of our Materia Medica and clinical experience.
This is when you have to make your own observations as to
what a potency is capable of curing and the reaction it
produces, which will eventually give you the experience you
require.

This can only come from inner confidence to prescribe,
which will in turn inspire your patient's confidence in you.
This volume is worthy of a place in any practitioner's
library, and if Hahnemann were alive today I feel he would
join me in congratulating the author of this book and
wishing him every success for the future.

Dr Kenneth Metson PhD.   September 1996

This is not intended as a definitive manual on the homœopathic treatment of HIV disease and AIDS, if there could be such a thing. Rather, it is a distillation of my experiences working at two of Europe's largest centres for people with these conditions.

Over the course of four years I treated some four hundred cases homœopathically. Despite intermittent burnout, depression and anxiety, this journey was like a rocket trip in terms of my own growth and understanding, not only of homœopathy, but about the role of healing in so-called 'terminal illnesses'.

I have added to my experiences the clinical research material of other authors, with their permission, where I have felt my own material is incomplete. I have also speculated (e.g. remedies I have not used but believe could be useful) where I have thought it appropriate.

All material presented should not be thought of as the final word on the matter but as stimulation for further research. Although this book is primarily intended for homœopaths, other therapists may find something of interest here. Also, the information presented here about AIDS may just as well apply to other immune disorders; indeed, all kinds of disease.

If it is true that every illness we suffer provides us with an opportunity to develop and grow, then AIDS has a unique gift in this regard.

I quote Edwin Steinbrecher:

"Many people think that taking responsibility for the total environment is a blame trip, but this is not so. We are truly responsible for the outer dream, but not to blame for it any more than we are to blame for the inner dream. We develop only as rapidly as we can accomplish the necessary psychological and physical changes. But, if you accept responsibility for what is happening in your world, then you can do something to change it in yourself. If you separate from your reality experience by thinking of it as unconnected to you, then there is nothing you can do to improve it." [1]

From the viewpoint of so-called 'classical' homœopathic prescribing some of the information in this book may seem revolutionary, if not disturbing! But I believe (and you will see) that in AIDS the highest degree of creativity is required from us as homœopaths and nothing less will do.

We have to develop the skill of lateral thinking. In short, we may have to break the 'rules'. But the rewards are tremendous, and positive results for our patients will always outweigh our own dogma (at least for most practitioners).

Perhaps it is the *spirit* of Samuel Hahnemann which is our best inspiration: keep learning, experiment and persevere.

Rx:	Prescription, remedy
>	Ameliorated, improved by,
<	Aggravated, made worse by,
+	Desires
Ø	Mother tincture
o.d.	One daily
b.d.	Twice daily
t.d.s.	Three times daily
N.B.W.S.	Never been well since
F.	Father
M.	Mother
F.F.	Fathers father
M.M.	Mothers mother
M.B.	Mothers brother etc

Introduction

AIDS is the disease of this age in the same way that
tuberculosis reflected the state of mankind in the early
years of this century. By this, I mean that AIDS perfectly
mirrors the concerns, fears and spiritual state of humanity
now, whether or not it appears to affect us personally.

AIDS is a world-wide phenomenon. It has caught the
imagination of vast numbers of people. It could even be
said to possess a kind of glamour - the images that are
evoked have a poetic quality to them (certainly in the West
people with AIDS are often seen as martyrs dying for a
cause). The recent 'Benetton' advertisement poster is a
good example. This depicts the moment of death of a man
with AIDS while his anguish-stricken parents look on. This
theme is echoed in numerous films, plays and books. The
association between well-meaning commercial sponsors
and celebrities with AIDS-related fund-raising projects may
have emphasised the illusion of glamour in the struggle
against insurmountable odds.

At the beginning of the AIDS scare, the status of gays in the
community plummeted to an all-time low because of the
fear that gay men were somehow threatening the very fabric
of society and were responsible for this 'plague'. At last,
people thought they had a valid reason for their prejudices
and could justify ostracising the gay section of society.
In response, though, the gay community were able to
demonstrate that they could be as responsible as anyone
in changing their sexual habits, and could, at the same time,
reclaim their self worth and integrity through fighting
against the prejudices which had always been part of the
gay / straight divide. Of course, AIDS does not only affect
the gay community, but it is perhaps meaningful that,
statistically speaking, all the main groups affected could be
perceived to have been abused either by themselves or

society². In this way AIDS has been a catalyst for the whole of society.

As an astrologer, in addition to being a homœopath, I was interested to learn that Pluto started its journey through Scorpio at the same time that AIDS became a sociological phenomenon, i.e. in 1984. Pluto in Scorpio, the sign of death and regeneration, indicates that power issues are foremost. The way that we individually and collectively use and abuse power concerning sex, the environment, death and disease has to be confronted. The dark side of our psyche, those 'neuroses' or taboos which have become separated from our consciousness will be brought to the surface to be examined and integrated - and these *are* the issues of our times. One could say that it is a case of 'regenerate or die'. One book written in the 1970's says that the transit of Pluto through Scorpio is the time in which there is the greatest danger of plague, famine, and atomic or biological warfare.³ Pluto concludes its sojourn in Scorpio in 1996.

AIDS could be said to provide a logical development in the history of illness and medicine. The collapse of the immune system begs for the deepest understanding of the nature of health and disease - and this presently eludes conventional medicine. Huge resources are being devoted to just one avenue of research - the search for a vaccine - based on the idea that the HIV virus is the sole or main cause of AIDS. Yet at present, none of the medical drugs being used transforms the course of the disease and a vaccine seems as far off a possibility as ever. Western medicine seems finally to have met its match. Most homœopaths think that the history of allopathic medicine is one of increasing suppression. If AIDS is the latest product of this process, then we can only recoil in dread at what the next step could be.

When AIDS first hit the headlines in around 1984 it quickly took on the mantle of 'most feared disease' which cancer had held for several decades. Like cancer, it was assumed that the prognosis for sufferers was automatically very poor. This resulted in a great deal of fear and caution amongst many alternative therapists. The other side of the coin, of course, was that as there was not much to lose, given the inadequacy of the conventional approach; we might as well 'have a go'.

At the two centres for AIDS where I have worked it quickly became apparent that the alternative therapies were the most popular services offered. Out of the therapies on offer, acupuncture, massage and other hands-on therapies seemed most in demand; whilst homœopathy, although not unpopular, did not seem to have quite the same draw.

There may be several reasons for this:

- confusion as to what exactly homœopathy is;
- the fact that homœopathy is frequently not as immediately gratifying as some other therapies;
- homœopathy requires more application on the part of the patient in terms of self exploration and discipline;
- being based on the prescription of pills brings it perilously close to the practice of conventional medicine, in the eyes of some patients.

Of course, as homœopaths we are also faced with difficult questions. For example, how do we counter the claim that HIV is the sole cause of AIDS? And if the HIV virus is unique among all of those that afflict mankind, how does that affect our ability to help our patients? These concerns may prove spurious but they have to be faced nevertheless. Looking positively, one great strength that homœopathy has in this situation, apart from the remedies themselves, is an alternative perspective on disease with which we can deconstruct the blame, victimisation and hopelessness which are such a large part of the AIDS scenario.

In At The Deep End

In 1990 I was invited to visit a centre for people with HIV/AIDS in South London . This led to my giving a talk on homœopathy at the Centre. I was apprehensive about meeting the very sick or those who were dying which I need not have been because my audience, in the event, seemed able-bodied, receptive and, one could say, quite normal.

At that time I was not confident of my ability to treat patients with a disease such as AIDS. It seemed too great a responsibility and, in truth, I felt somewhat inadequate.

Nevertheless, in spite of my doubts, one month later I saw my first patient. Here is his case:

Case: 26.7.90   Male 30 years of age.
He had recently undergone three operations for bowel cancer; these had left him with an open wound in his rectum which bled on passing stool and was very painful. He had frequent rectal herpes; shingles earlier in the year and a number of ear infections. He was breathless after walking only a short distance since pneumonia in January. He had lost three stone in just over 12 months and was extremely weak.
He was irritable and edgy, but open with his feelings; he was affectionate and sympathetic. When he felt unwell he was fiercely independent and wanted to be alone. He was frightened of dying and of disability.
His childhood had been very unhappy; his parents didn't want him, and sent him to boarding school. His father was violent, an alcoholic and a transvestite; and he hated his son's homosexuality.

Medical drugs he was taking were:
Acyclovir (herpes), AZT (HIV inhibitor), Fluconazole (thrush), Pentamidine, (PCP), Imodium (diarrhœa),

Gastrocoat (antacid), Naproxen (anti-inflammatory), DF118 (painkillers), Lactulose, (for the side effects of DF118), multivitamins, chemotherapy.

Medical History:
Born prematurely; weighed two pounds at birth. Neonatal jaundice, whooping cough, glandular fever, kidney failure, appendicitis, peritonitis, multiple pneumonia, asthma, tonsillitis, ulcerative colitis. Vaccinations: BCG, cholera, typhoid, yellow fever, smallpox, diphtheria.

Family History:
Father: hermaphrodite; gall bladder and part of colon removed; cysts.
Mother: hepatitis, rheumatoid arthritis
Maternal grandfather: died in Nazi concentration camp
Paternal grandmother: dementia, high blood pressure.
Paternal grandfather: died of cancer
Sister: Cancer of cervix
Brother: Cirrhosis of liver, alcoholism.

After I had recovered from the shock of case-taking I took a deep breath and got on with the job. I realised that this was no ordinary classical case (!) and would probably need frequent change and repetition of remedies.

I recommended that he give up as many of the drugs as was comfortable and prescribed the following:

Rx: *Carcinosin* 30 once a day for five days;
Arnica / Hypericum 30 three times daily; (tds)
Echinacea Ø, Calendula Ø, Malandrinum Ø and
Pyrogen 6 tds

Carcinosin was for the general emotional and physical suppression and history of trauma, plus a history of cancer. (I have found that repetition of the remedy is essential in excessively drugged cases).
Arnica and *Hypericum* was to help the healing following his operations.

Echinacea Ø, Calendula Ø, Malandrinum Ø and *Pyrogen* 6
I decided to experiment with this last combination as a
general blood purifier. *Malandrinum* is known to clear the
remnants of cancerous deposits.

2.8.90 A week later. He was sleeping better and was
less irritable. His rectum continued to be very painful
where the sphincter had been cut. He still felt afraid of
death and being alone. He had a strong desire for cold
drinks.

Rx: *Phosphorus* 30 once daily for a week
          Staphysagria 200 as needed for pain.

He presented a *Phosphorus* constitutional picture. His
rectum did not seem to be healing as one might have
wished so *Staphysagia* fitted the invasive aspect of the
surgery, excessive pain and the affinity to the sphincters.

9.8.90 Another week on, his rectum was healing fast,
and the pain had lessened.
His T4 (lymphocyte) count was up 250%, from 50 to
186. He felt much better in himself and more
contented.
He had nausea, worse between 11 pm and 1.30 am
and accompanied by profuse sweats on his forehead,
difficult breathing, and heat.
He was vomiting and had eructations of bile which
were better for small amounts of water. He had rectal
herpes and fissures.

Rx: *Arnica* 10M, *Carcinosin* 10M, *Staphysagria* 10M
          Tuberculinum 1M , *AZT* 30
          (*Veratrum Album* 30 and *Nitricum Acidum* 6 as
          required)

Encouraged by the patient's positive reaction I decided to
repeat some of the previous remedies in higher potencies.
Tuberculinum followed naturally after *Carcinosin* and
Phosphorus. Prescribing *AZT* was an attempt to clear any
toxicity of this drug from the system.

I will often combine an acute prescription with one for the chronic state. Thus the *Veratrum Album* fitted the nausea picture whilst the *Nitricum Acidum* was for the rectal fissures. In AIDS I believe one often has to 'throw' remedies at patients without being too concerned about the niceties of Kentian philosophy. The situation is frequently complex and changes quickly and one has to keep apace.

The patient displayed, at this time, a distinct change of attitude to his condition and to his doctors. He apparently challenged them with an article from *The Lancet* on the side effects of AZT and demanded to know why they had not told him about these. Until then he had been a mild accepting person, not wanting to cause any trouble.

6.9.90 After the above remedies he developed headaches and then - possibly - a mild case of meningitis. These soon passed and after that he felt great, happy and contented, and looked well. His rectal pain had subsided, and his wound had almost healed. His nausea and vomiting were gone.

I would dearly love to be able to say that following homœopathic treatment this patient wandered into the sunset, happy and healthy. What happened in reality gave the story a strange, ironic twist. The patient, now well enough to travel the world (unimaginable in his original state), met his death at the hands of a murderer on a Mediterranean island.

Nevertheless, it should be said that this patient had made great headway in a short space of time, showing me that homœopathy had enormous potential in the treatment of AIDS.

Taking The Case

"The moment I recognise the problem as factual I cannot help the patient." [4]

Raymond Charles Barker

In AIDS we often see a confused symptom picture. Clear remedy pictures are not the order of the day. There is likely to be a complex background of trauma, illness and suppression; severe physical pathology, both acute and chronic; several active miasms; frequent acute episodes; much drug treatment; depleted vital energy and low expectations. The medical and drug history alone can take thirty or forty minutes to establish.

I have found it most useful when taking or studying a case to consider the following areas:

- **Aetiology**

- **Emotional traumas, especially those of childhood**

- **Miasmatic tendencies**

- **Organ weaknesses and affinities**

- **Constitutional type**

There are various important points which need to be investigated:

- **What was the patient's reaction to testing HIV+?**
- **Their attitude towards HIV and AIDS and their health in general.**
- **What drugs are they taking, prescribed or recreational, and what is their attitude towards these?**
- **Medical history including vaccinations, drugs, venereal diseases (hepatitis, gonorrhoea, non-specific urethritis (NSU), syphilis, herpes).**
- **Details of their childhood, especially if traumatic, in as much detail as time permits.**
- **Family history, including mental disorder, alcoholism and violence.**
- **Possible aetiologies, e.g. grief, disappointments, loss of vital fluids (seminal fluid, perspiration, blood), blood transfusions, candidiasis.**

From this information the next task is to sift through and choose the most relevant and significant factors and themes, which will usually be those that most limit the patient's ability to function. The most limiting factors should be assessed and treated first. Where the patient feels the most pain (mental or physical) is often the best guide. Extreme physical pain has to be dealt with early on, and sometimes independently from the rest of the case as it will often prevent progress on other levels. Sometimes one has to consider treating the disease first as, in many cases, the constitutional remedy serves merely to strengthen the individual but does not cure.

One has to make decisions about which drugs are likely to interfere with treatment (see 'drugs' section), any lifestyle changes which may be necessary - I have, for example, seen patients who indulge in casual sex and become re-infected with gonorrhœa whilst receiving homœopathic treatment.

Prescribing And Case Management

"Very notable surgeons... and others are at times condescendingly hopeful that we may look forward to the day when 'a remedy for cancer' will be discovered. Whatever knowledge such people possess, there are two things of which they know nothing real, viz., cancer, and the modes of action of remedies in cancer and cancerous diseases. You might as well try to grow potatoes in a field consisting of one chemical element instead of ordinary humus.... This running after one remedy for any disease of complex nature is simple ignorance of fundamental principles and bars the road to progress. Cancer is a chain of links, and each kind has links of different nature and each link is a biological process. And you are going to alter all that with 'a' remedy? It is absolutely unthinkable, and has no parallel in physio-biological phenomena." [5]

James Compton Burnett
(for 'cancer' read 'AIDS')

The qualities required in the effective homœopathic treatment of HIV/AIDS are flexibility, practicality and creativity. The ability to think laterally is a distinct advantage.

There is no substitute for a good knowledge of materia medica, including small remedies, organ remedies, various permutations of mineral salts, sarcodes, tautopathic remedies and, of course, polychrests. One also should be well versed in anatomy, physiology and the pathological processes, especially those related to the organs and endocrine glands. Although routine prescribing usually fails, a good knowledge of therapeutics (prescribing for the disease process) can prove invaluable. I cannot emphasise enough the importance of exploring the byways of homœopathy rather in addition to the well trodden polychrest route.

As many AIDS cases do not display the simple 'classical' picture I find it helpful to identify the different foci of the case and if there is no single remedy which covers the totality I would look at multiple remedies which cover the presenting picture.

I find it sometimes helps to set myself a target when I first see a patient; for example, if there is a powerful emotional state I recognise the importance of dealing with this quickly; likewise with pain.

One of the great limitations of so-called classical prescribing is the fixed idea that there is one remedy and one remedy *only* which can work at any one time. I have found this to be a limiting concept in the treatment of some cases of AIDS. There are all kinds of approaches, varying with each case. Someone once said that a chaotic disease may take chaotic prescribing. Certainly an 'elegant' prescription is not always necessary in these types of cases.

As a general rule, be conscious of which level of awareness you are working with in each patient. At any given time in the treatment schedule, there are different healing tasks for us to accomplish. One of the most common mistakes I have found in homœopathic treatment is prescribing at the wrong level. Some patients are straightforward in that the disease process starts in the mind and comes down, so to speak, in a direct line into the body. It is these that simply need the 'constitutional' remedy. Other patients may be too anxious, grief-stricken or tense, so that they are not 'vibrating' on the level of the constitutional remedy, even though that may seem indicated, and these are the patients that will need 'warming-up' remedies.

Sometimes the most deep-acting remedy is not appropriate. It may be that a more acute or superficial remedy would work better by opening up and preparing the patient for the deeper or 'soul' remedies at a later stage. Flower essences may be useful in this connection as they will often smooth the way.

More than one remedy may be indicated at any one time because each patient has different dimensions that interact and exist alongside each other. Obviously, in AIDS we are frequently dealing with patients who are extremely anxious. If we prescribe for the anxiety in an acute sense it is possible to make headway quickly.

Generally speaking, patients with HIV/AIDS need particular attention and emotional support and may usefully be seen by the practitioner more often than would normally be the case; possibly every day or two in very acute cases to two to four weekly in less pressing cases.

In many cases I have found it necessary to prescribe more often; following the progress of the case carefully and supporting with remedies at each point. This is especially important at the beginning of treatment when the confidence of the patient is often fragile and one needs to demonstrate quite quickly the efficacy of the treatment. In my experience giving different remedies at short intervals very rarely, if ever, has the disastrous effects predicted by Kent and his followers.

In acute conditions do not wait too long after prescribing if there is no discernible improvement. Reassess the case and prescribe again.

It should be emphasised that treating AIDS is often very different from the more leisurely pace normally experienced in our practices.

Because of the nature of AIDS which usually consists of a chronic state with numerous acute 'flare-ups', it is important to address all of the different phases, giving acute remedies interspersed with more chronic treatment as and when required.

The cases which prove the most intractable and need the most work are often those where the patients are taking powerful or large amounts of allopathic drugs. Ideally, such cases would be seen on a daily basis in a hospital-type environment which, of course, is not often practicable.

Kentian	Eclectic
One remedy at a time based on totality of symptoms. Assumes only one process in operation at any one time.	Concept of layers or levels. One or more remedies may be prescribed sequentially. Use of drainage, organ support and complementary remedies.
Allow remedy to run its full course before re-prescribing.	Build on progress already achieved. Frequent prescriptions OK where appropriate. Treat certain aggravations, acute flare ups.
Never change remedy where there has been improvement.	Repeat remedy where appropriate or prescribe for new picture or different aspect of case.
Lesions are part of totality and much be prescribed on as such.	Lesions may be prescribed for separately where they have a picture of their own or using therapeutics
Nosodes should never be repeated at quick succession.	Nosodes used freely, sequentially, in acutes etc.

The Layers Model

"There are several cases of disease in which the administration of a double remedy is perfectly Homœopathic and truly rational; where for instance, each of two medicines appears suited for the case of disease, but each from a different side; or where the case of disease depends on more than one of the three radical causes of chronic diseases discovered by me, as when in addition to psora we have to do with syphilis or sycosis also." [6]

Samuel Hahnemann

I have found the idea of layers of pathology highly useful in treating HIV and AIDS. As I have already said , I often find that to prescribe on more than one layer simultaneously may give more thorough results. Conventional homœopathic wisdom, though accepting the existence of 'layers' of pathology as set out by Eizayaga,[7] dictates that only one layer at a time should be treated. I do not deny the effectiveness of this in many cases but I would also add that it is possible to prescribe for more than one layer at a time, especially where there is much 'inertia' through complex aetiologies and drugging, to take an example.

We have to match our prescription not just on symptom similarity but with the intensity of the energy of the case. Thus, we may need to address the case from different angles using more than one remedy.

In sequential prescribing we identify the different layers or aspects of the case and prescribe a different remedy for each of these layers. These are prescribed in sequence, usually in single high potency doses, spaced from a few minutes to a day apart. Another way would be for such remedies to be alternated on a regular basis.

It should be pointed out that this approach is not a short cut to avoid the discipline of learning materia medica or a deep perception of the case. If anything it is quite the reverse: it allows us to perceive the case as it truly is unhindered by rigid dogma.

Patient who have profound and complex emotional pathology may benefit from sequential prescribing. We may perceive a *Calcarea Carbonica* constitutional picture overlaid with *Carcinosin* (emotional suppression) and *Aurum* (suicidal tendencies). In this type of case *Carcinosin* and *Calcarea Carbonica* could be prescribed in high potency single doses, together with *Aurum* 200 which may be taken as and when required. In appropriate cases this may give dramatically positive results. It should be noted that homœopathic remedies may be used in a similar way to flower essences, to deal with crystallised psychological blocks - which may be likened to emotional tumours. Each remedy thus addresses a particular aspect of the whole.

Here is a case which illustrates this approach:

Case: Male 30 yrs. HIV+ for 2 yrs
Fatigue. Legs weak
Night sweats - all over body
Itchy, scaly rash - forehead, face < washing
Feet burning hot in bed which he sticks out of covers.
Suppresses anger leading to depression and anxiety.
Wants to be alone. Sympathy <.
Recently, a man sexually interfered with him - feels angry, tight chest
Does not cry easily; cuts off from his emotions.
Remembers little about childhood. Abuse?
Gay.
Most of life has felt suicidal. Wild as teenager.
Fears: death, pain, dependency, rape, big dogs.
Averse cold, damp.
Sleepless 'thinking about old stuff'
Very high sex drive

Appetite: good   + bread, potatoes
                        < eggs
Medical History: Chicken pox, epilepsy (aged two)
Chest infections. Anal warts operated on 3 yrs ago
Drugs: Septrin, Codeine phosphate, Cortisone cream
Patient has had many drugs, recreational and medical,
in last year.
Family History: Mother- TB; Father- high blood
pressure; MF- died bowel cancer;
MM- died bowel cancer; MB- circulatory problems.

Rx: *Septrin* 30 alternating with *Sulphur* 30 once daily
    for three days, then split doses on consecutive
    days: *Carcinosin* 10M, *Tuberculinum* 10M,
    Staphysagria 10M.

Here, I saw someone with vague physical symptoms, much
suppression and a great deal of emotional trauma. Three
remedies (*Carc., Tub.,* and *Staph.*) may be identified in this
case and they will all work at different levels. I decided to
use this combination to try to clarify the picture and used
Septrin and *Sulphur* as a detoxifying combination.

At 2 months
Night sweats >
Remembered that Father had sexually abused
him and the terror this had caused.
Gingivitis - bleeding, receding gums.
Nightmares - wakes in a cold sweat, terrified.
Wants to be alone.
Wants to cry but cannot.
Holding on to anger.

Rx: *Stramonium* 10M followed by *Natrum Muriaticum*
    200, 1M, 10M the following day; then *Mercurius* 30
    alternating with *Sulphur* 30 once daily for 10 days

The previous presciption has unlocked emotional feelings
and memories which had been suppressed. I felt this to be
a good sign.
One could argue that I should have perhaps continued the

same remedies but I followed Compton Burnett's advice on how ringing-the-changes with remedies sometimes gives better results. Again, all the above remedies can be seen to be indicated: *Stramonium* for the terror; *Natrum Muriaticum* for the held-in grief; *Mercurius* for the gingivitis (perhaps, constitutionally as well); continuing, also, with the *Sulphur* for the detox.

Obviously, a great deal of intuition and a clinical knowledge of how the remedies act goes into a prescription such as that above. In many cases I do not believe that there is only one correct prescription. The cases I cite offer one solution to a problem but I am sure there will be others. Sometimes the rationale may seem difficult to grasp but I hope these cases will, at least, suggest ideas and provide stimulation for your own cases.

At 3 months
Gums >. After remedies developed flu.
Now more energy.
Cough - green/yellow expectoration < on waking
Emotionally feels good; started an evening class.
Hot feet at night. Itchy patches on face.
Desires chocolate

Rx: *Sulphur* 10M single dose and
          Pulsatilla 30 once daily for five days.

The case seems to be 'simplifying'. *Sulphur* still seemed indicated on the basis of the physicals and *Pulsatilla* was given as an acute support remedy for the cough.

At 4 months
Felt really well - 'magical time'. Mentally and physically cleared .
'Feeling better and better.'
Still getting nightmares about sexual abuse. Wakes terrified with sweating.
Gingivitis with salivation, receding gums, bad breath.

Rx: *Syphilinum* 10M; *Stramonium* 10M; *Opium* 10M; *Mercurius* 10M; on consecutive nights.

Again, it could be argued that one should wait whilst there is improvement taking place. But I have found that in practice this is often not necessary and one can build on the improvement already achieved by re-prescribing. This is not always so but more especially in cases where there is a strong emotional element.

The case seemed to show an underlying syphilitic tendency, given the amount of sexual abuse, thus *Syphilinum*. *Stramonium* and *Opium* often work well together. They are especially useful where there is a powerful trauma element with much fear and/or terror. *Mercurius* reinforces the *Syphilinum*. I decided on 10M potency for its powerful effect at the deepest levels of the being.

At 5¹/₂ months
Feels really well. Nightmares have stopped.
No gingivitis.

Rx: None

As with many patients who are HIV+, he did not continue the treatment. However, I recently (July 1996) happened to meet this patient again and he seemed well.

This approach may also suit victims of shock and trauma. I recall a patient who had been mugged and had received a stab wound in the back. Two days after the incident I prescribed *Aconite, Opium, Arnica* and *Stramonium* 200 alternating (there was no time for subtle remedy differentiation) plus *Hypercal* ointment to dress the wound. He returned the following week. In his words, 'the wound just closed up' and the symptoms of shock had completely dispersed.

In practice, many of the objections to this way of prescribing are unfounded.[8] Two common objections can be answered as follows:

· **It is impossible to tell which remedy has worked.**
You do not need to know which remedy is working to get a positive result. The next time patients come to you they will be in a different state and you will be able to reassess the situation and prescribe either one or more remedies accordingly. Sometimes, we have to decide which is more important: the wellbeing of the patient or the education of the homœopath.

· **Surely the remedies interfere with one another.**
In my experience, the remedies do not have a negative interference effect on each other. In practice, after one or two treatments the picture often consolidates and a more 'classical' picture appears which can be approached in a more traditional way. The object should be to use what works and in AIDS cases there is urgency. However well indicated the remedy and however philosophically sound the thinking, in my experience a single dose of the simillimum may do very little.

Certain people do not, it has to be said, respond so well to multi-remedy prescribing. These tend to be the more frail or sensitive types who may aggravate. These cases often need a single remedy prescribed in a low or LM potency. If, by chance, there is a bad aggravation from the use of more than one remedy, a reassessment of the original case may be required. In such cases you may find one remedy which will cover the totality. However, it is helpful to discern between frailty and simple low energy. The latter, in my experience, can take high potencies with no ill effects.

Sometimes one has to identify what is important in a case, addressing that and, for the time being, ignoring the rest of the case. For example, where a patient has an inflamed liver with weakness, the liver problem may be the outstanding symptom (perhaps requiring liver drainage), and in this kind of case, the miasmatic history and the constitution should 'take a back seat' until the liver problem is under control, when the rest of the case can then be assessed and treated more confidently.

When there is a desperate search for a single remedy (the 'Holy Grail' method, as I call it), as if that were the only way to prescribe, often there is a good deal of fear about giving the wrong remedy. We can easily become obsessed about this and become, in a sense, paralysed. This, in itself, can lead to excessive caution and less effective homœopathy than is possible. I find it helpful to remember that what ever my prescription I will receive important information about the case on the next session. So, rather than a 'right versus wrong' view, there is, in reality, a continual feedback from which we can learn.

Sequential and multi-layer prescribing is not for every patient (or every practitioner) but for those homœopaths who want to open their minds it can be a very useful addition to the repertoire.

Here is another case showing the use of multi-layer prescribing

Case: Male 28 yrs HIV+
Always had depression but < since one year
Feels lonely and sad. Generally < alone, night.
Feels inferior to others. One year ago was suicidal.
Fears rejection, alone, dying alone, cats, insects.
Had a relationship with woman for six years but she couldn't cope with his HIV+ status. She left him. As a child much violence from stepfather towards himself and mother. This made him angry and scared. Mother and stepfather were alcoholic. There are parts of his childhood about which he cannot remember anything (sexual abuse?) Very hard to cry. Suppresses feelings. Very frightened of own anger. He either backs off or lets people walk all over him. Was violent in teenage years. Would start fights with anyone.

Difficult sleep. Worries about finances, daughter etc.
For three months - night sweats (sour).
Persistent diarrhœa < eating. Drives him out of bed in
morning.
Craves: Spicy, milk, chicken, salt.
Drinks 4 pints icy drinks per day
Feet always hot esp. in bed

Medical History: Shingles, many accidents and
concussion. Lots of minor chest infections and
antibiotics.
Drugs: Used to take heroin, valium, marijuana for
twelve years. Gave them up three years ago. Then
relapsed one year ago but has been off everything for
ten weeks.
Family History: M- Alcoholic, takes drugs, bulimia, TB,
suicidal.; F- Suicidal, died heart attack; MF- murdered;
MM- died cancer; FF- mentally ill; MB-killed by train

Rx: *Sulphur* 30 od for 3 days then *Stramonium* 10M,
       Tuberculinum 10M, *Syphilinum* 10M on consecutive
       days and *Coffea* 30 nightly as required for
       sleeplessness.

This is the kind of case where the above method of
prescribing comes into its own. There is a whole complex
of symptoms and layers of pathology, and I have found that
prescribing multiple remedies based on the different layers
floods the system with energy. There were strong
tubercular and syphilitic indications combined with acute
terror (*Stramonium*). *Sulphur*, again, is indicated as a general
'blood purifier'.

One week later
The patient has made a dramatic improvement:
'like I've shed a skin'. Sleeping 10 hours a night.
'People cannot stop me from talking. I'm walking
around with a bounce in my step'.
No loneliness or sadness. Diarrhœa much >.
Feet still hot. Profuse night sweats.

Rx: *Sulphur* 1M to carry on the detoxification

4 Months later
Feels generally very well. Has a new girlfriend.
Hot feet, sweating and painful sinuses at night.
T4 count now 946 (100% better than first consultation).

Rx: *Sulphur* 10M + *Mercurius* 30 bd for 7 days

Sulphur seems to be this patient's constitutional remedy.
Mercury fitted the other physicals and complements
Sulphur well. I have found the idea of one dose of a high
potency remedy, say the constutional, together with
repeated doses of a lower potency support remedy works
well.

Question: was the dramatic leap in the T4 cell count due to
the remedies or his falling in love? (I have noticed a similar
effect in other patients).

So, how does Hering's Law apply, for example, in the cases
we are discussing here? Hering wrote his law from his own
experience - it was not written in stone. Sometimes we see
Hering's Law in operation and sometimes not.

I believe that we all know when a patient is getting better
from their increased vitality, sense of control, well being
and increased ability to function in the world. Often we
see a clarification or focusing of the picture as the patient
gets better, as the vital force becomes more integrated and
this is the true measure of whether we have been
successful in our efforts.

Aetiologies

In many cases, as we know, there is a direct connection between a past trauma of some kind - grief, violent attack, unresolved illness, drugging or vaccination - and the present state of ill-health. For example, one patient had been mugged in the street and had never been well since that time. In spite of being HIV+ for some years, it was this event which was the crucial trigger. It is sometimes necessary to do some detective work to uncover hidden aetiologies which may seem minor to the patient. One AIDS patient was responding well to treatment although his energy was still somewhat low and he had chronic enlarged tonsils. It was only after his vaccination history came to light that I realised that *Thuja* was indicated and, indeed, this helped greatly

Many patients with AIDS have one or more indirect or long-term aetiologies in the form of certain family or life situations which have contributed to a decline in health over a period of time.

Constitutional Prescribing

This assumes an orderly progression of disease from the mental and emotional levels of the being to the physical. Here, conflict arises between so-called 'classical' and 'non-classical' homœopaths, because to treat the local symptoms of disease or the physical organs is considered to result in suppression. I have not found this to be the case in practice. I usually find constitutional prescribing useful once the strands of the case have come together to form a coherent whole. Often, this is not the situation at the beginning of treatment and it takes a period of 'clarifying' treatment to reach this point. It is, of course, worthwhile for the patient to receive constitutional treatment but many HIV / AIDS patients are of a restless, tubercular nature and do not continue their treatment.

Drainage, Low Potency Support and Organ Remedies

These combinations can be prescribed prior to, or along side, the main constitutional or miasmatic remedies. Where there is organ dysfunction or congestion which hinders the eliminative functions, the indicated, deep-acting constitutional remedy may be blocked in its action and a severe aggravation may result. The indicated drainage remedy or remedies improve the function of the organ, thus paving the way for the action of the deeper constitutional remedy. Organ remedies are, therefore, homœopathic at the level of the organ. They are prescribed in low potency repeated doses (usually two to three times a day).

Some interesting remedies/ combinations:

*Chelidonium / Hydrastis Canadensis / Carduus Marianus*6x

- general liver drainage

Chelidonium / Quercus Glandium / Nux Vomica 6x

- liver drainage for alcoholics; helps to lessen the craving.

Chelidonium / Hydrastis / Nux Vomica 6x

- liver drainage after much drugging.

Thyroidinum / Fucus Vesiculosus/ Iodum 6

- thyroid support

Pulsatilla / Sepia / Lilium Tigrinum / Caulophyllum / Fraxinus Americanus 6 - brings back absent menses

Calcarea Arsenicosum 6

- pancreas and kidney drainage (with much anxiety)

As the organ improves on a physical level the mental and emotional states of the patient may worsen. This is where the patient has, for instance, 'held' stress in the organ and as treatment procedes this manifests itself in the higher spheres. Essentially, a return of old symptoms.

Flower Essences

These include: Bach, Australian Bush, Californian and Bailey essences. They are useful in the following situations:

- Prior to homœopathic treatment where there is a deeply ingrained attitude or belief structure. Here such prescribing can ease resistance to change.

- To support the patient when there is a clearly positive response to homœopathic prescribing but which brings strong emotions to the surface or initiates a process of emotional or spiritual change.

- Where there is a strong attachment to a maintaining cause such as a relationship from which the patient is ready to move on but lacks the courage to do so.

Some flower essences worth exploring:

Gorse (Bach): Despair of recovery

Sweet Chestnut (Bach): Anguish: 'dark night of the soul'

Rock Rose (Bach): Terror

Wild Rose (Bach): Apathy, resignation

Walnut (Bach): Protection from powerful influences during big life changes.

Self-Heal (Californian): Finding inner motivation to be well

Spruce (Californian): Detox after chemo- and radio-therapy

Billy Goat Plum (Australian Bush): Self disgust, physical loathing

Macrocarpa (Australian Bush): Exhausted, low immunity, convalescence

Spinifex (Australian Bush): Feeling victim to illness, herpes.

Auto-isopathy and Sarcodes

Prescribing the patient's own blood in potency has seen to yield positive, if not dramatic, results and is certainly worth considering, although in some cases homœopathy can be less effective when the *similar* becomes *identical.* Urine therapy (i.e. the patient's own) has also been seen to be useful. One patient applied urine topically to his Karposi's Sarcoma lesions.

Some interesting material has arisen with regards to *Thymus Gland* (see Materia Medica section). The full range of sarcodes is under-used, in my estimation. More clinical research and provings need to be done on remedies (including mental/emotional states) that include, for example: *Pancreas, Liver, Hypothalamus, Pituitary, Urinum Humanum, Thalamus, Cortisone, A.C.T. Hormone,* etc.

Nosodes

Nosodes can be used to clear the picture. They are often needed more frequently in HIV/AIDS than other types of case because of the intense and often deeply ingrained spiritual pathology that can often be traced through the family history. In terms of miasmatic susceptibility AIDS is a product of all the miasms, often combined: psora, sycosis, syphilis, cancer. I have found three main miasmatic 'pathways' or sequential states:

• *Carcinosin - Medorrhinum - Thuja*
• *Carcinosin - Tuberculinum - Syphilinum*
• *Carcinosin - Tuberculinum - Thuja*

There are of course others. These can be prescribed in sequence, on successive days, for example. The choice of nosodes depends on the prominent miasms in the medical and/or family history, and may have the effect of clearing the picture and raising the energy level very quickly.

For example, take a theoretical case: A man has had a very traumatic childhood with a great deal of emotional suppression. In his twenties he had several bouts of gonorrhoea and much dope; so he is spaced out, feels detached from himself and society and has marked mood swings. Now he sweats profusely, has stomach ulcers and salivates onto his pillow at night. We could prescribe in the following way: *Carcinosin* 10M (Monday), *Medorrhinum* 10M (Tuesday), *Thuja* 10M (Wednesday) followed by *Mercurius* 30 twice daily for 5 days. The *Carcinosin* relates to the history of emotional suppression; *Medorrhinum* and *Thuja* covers the sycotic aspects of gonorrhoea and recreational drug use and the *Mercurius* will deal with the more immediate physical pathology. The prescription of three high potency remedies in sequence can flood the patient with energy and this has a tremendous positive effect.

In a simpler case, one might prescribe the underlying miasmatic nosode followed by the constitutional remedy in either a single dose or repeated low potency doses. There are many ways to the same goal.

The nosodes should not only be thought of for the chronic state; some of the most dramatic results have been gained from using the nosodes in acute conditions.
Apart from the standard nosodes we may consider unusual nosodes such as:

Candida Albicans	*Toxoplasma Gondii*
Cryptosporidium	*Cytomegalovirus*
Epstein-Barr virus	*Pneumocystis Carinii*
Herpes Virus	*Mycobacteria*
Cryptococci	*Coxsackie Virus*
Leprominium	*Malaria*
Typhoidinum	

Plus a myriad of *Streptococci* and *Staphylococci*

These can often have the effect of breaking down the individual toxins, whilst appropriate drainage or constitutional remedies will encourage their elimination.

The following case demonstrates the use of multiple nosodes in a complex situation:

Case: 3.12.92 Male: 39 yrs of age.

Haemophiliac all his life. Now HIV+
Left knee hot and painful and with haemorrhage into knee capsule. < cold, damp. > continued motion
Feels hot at night and sticks feet out of covers.
Much < stuffy room, hot weather;
Swollen glands in nape of neck and under arms
Has regular factor 8 (clotting agent) transfusions
Urine dark, very strong smell.
Easily haemorrhages in knees, left ankle, right testicle.
Once a month spontaneous ejaculation of blood.
Desires sweets, cheese, milk, < meat, much < alcohol
Quite undisciplined, untidy. Says he is a bit of a recluse.
Angry with (dominant) mother. She treats him like a child. Cannot express how he feels to her, suppresses his feelings. Says he feels as if he is dying.

Rx :   *Carcinosin* 10M, (Mondays) *Tuberculinum* 10M, (Tuesdays) *Syphilinum* 10M (Wednesdays); repeated for four weeks. Also *Phosphorus* 6 and *Thymus Gland* 6 twice daily alternating for a week.

I used consecutive nosodes to help clear the miasmatic picture, to act as a 'bomb', to bring in a great deal of energy. *Phosphorus* was given on the basis of his sympathetic nature and the haemophiliac tendency to bleed easily; also on a more constitutional level. *Thymus Gland* was used as an organ support remedy .

4.2.93
After remedies felt really good. However, father died two weeks ago. Now bleeding badly in testicle. Very upset. Took *Staphysagria* for emotional reaction which

> testicle. Testes very swollen, throbbing, bruised.
Haematuria when aroused if doesn't ejaculate. Very
tired last couple of weeks.

Rx: Repeat of last prescription.

The previous prescription had done what was required but
the patient had experienced a trauma which had set him
back. Here, we see the need to remain flexible and to
prescribe as frequently as necessary, following closely the
patient's life problems when they arise.

10.4.93
Felt fine after last remedies.
Sore throat, neck glands swollen.
Bleeding from right testicle, swollen, tight, hot.
Has had a lot of factor 8 transfusions.
Sweating a lot at night. Sometimes smelling badly.
Sleepless 2-3 am with burning in chest.
Patient is rocking on his chair in consultation room.

Rx: *Mercurius Corrosivus 200* as required.

The last symptom which gave me the clue to this
prescription was the patient's rocking, but I also realised
that although there were good indications for *Mercurius Sol.*
the picture was more violent, with the emphasis on
spontaneous bleeding.

21.6.93
Last remedies worked well for bleeding. Felt very
good. Recently had a typhoid vaccination. Aching arm,
sore axilla, aching all over. Feels body 'not here' -
numb. Chilly, difficult breathing - throat swollen.

Rx: *Thuja* 10M

Thuja for ill effects of vaccination.

14.8. 93
> then < Really tired. Mind sluggish
Perspiration on face on waking

Rx: *Carcinosin* 10M followed by *Silica* 10M.

Thuja did not act deeply enough, so I returned to *Carcinosin* and added *Silica* to give the patient 'grit' to throw off the vaccination. This strategy worked.

31.5.94
5 weeks ago - cough started, < pollution, night.
Expectoration green/yellow. Took antibiotics. Led to bowel inflammation, itching of skin.
Swollen tonsils < right side.
Aversion to tea, desires Coca Cola
Constriction of chest. Cough < talking loudly.
Congested right lung. Regurgitates food on coughing.

Rx: *Phosphorus* 30

6.9.94
Piles - sore, burning, itchy, bleeding. > warm bath.
Constipation < coffee. Knees painful. Mother-in-law died to whom he was close. Did a great deal of caring, lot of tears. Difficult to cry. Can't relax.

Rx: *Causticum* 10M

Notice that as the case progressed, the intervals between treatment became longer, and, at publication of this book (Oct. 1996), the patient is doing well. Another remedy worth considering for the acute bleeding episodes of haemophiliacs is *Crotalus Horridus* (recommended by Kenneth Metson).

The Nature Of The Work

*"You must have perfect confidence in yourself, at the
same time instilling this confidence into your patient,
assuring him that you are going to eliminate his pain
and trouble. Assume that calm assurance of power. Do
not allow the slightest doubt to interfere with you and
your patient. You must act in a positive manner. The
more positive you are the more power you will generate.
These fundamental principles in the art of healing are
essential to your success, because they give you that
awareness, that confidence in the power to heal."* [9]

Murdo MacDonald-Bayne

Both the physical and emotional aspects of HIV/AIDS create
special demands upon the practitioner. It can be exhausting
treating people who have a fear and a deep belief that they
are dying, and the practitioner will need to find an inner
strength to avoid colluding with that prognosis. The
rewards, however, of helping patients to a different view of
their life and health in general are great indeed. Once life
and health are viewed in a spirit of exploration rather than
in simple terms of 'cured' or 'terminal' then a great step
forward has been made. In such a context fear often
provides the greatest obstacle. I have found enthusiasm for
the work an effective antidote to some of these negative
aspects, as it is often infectious! Interestingly, the word
'enthusiasm' is derived from the Greek meaning 'full of the
God-spirit'.

When one takes on working with people with so-called life
threatening diseases, it quickly becomes obvious that the
work is a continuing challenge and requires constant
commitment. One has always to be able to think on one's
feet with regards to the purely homœopathic elements of
treatment, as the patient's requirements are constantly

shifting. Having said that, it is my firm belief (and borne out by my experience) that with good homœopathic treatment we can justifiably expect to prolong life indefinitely for those patients who are asymptomatic. This can also be true for those in the initial stages of AIDS where remarkable recoveries are possible. For those who are more severely ill the future is perhaps less certain and will probably depend on the amount of conventional drugging together with the degree of strength of will to live, but in these cases often the quality of life can be improved at the very least.

Treating the person, not the virus, may seem obvious to a homœopath given the philosophy on which our science is based but it is sometimes more difficult in the HIV/AIDS situation, taking into account the conditioning of our culture. Many patients depersonalise themselves, they *become* the label and forget their human integrity; the virus becomes all-powerful in their minds and this in turn further undermines the immune system. However, by emphasising the importance of the immune system and homœopathy's ability to stimulate its functioning, together with good homœopathic prescribing, we can help patients to regain a more balanced perspective.

It becomes obvious that there is a need to educate as well as to prescribe, this is probably true for all types of patient, but even more so for those with HIV diagnosis. Creating a new context for the disease may be just what is needed to allow the person to feel safe and empowered, acting as a balance to the conventional model of health which often seems to have the opposite effect.

Many patients have low expectations of the benefits of treatment, indeed of life in general. They often perceive alternative medicine in terms of mild symptomatic relief or for relaxation purposes, but nothing deeper. Some patients even confess to not expecting to live beyond the age of thirty or thirty-five years.

Education and counselling is a crucial part of the treatment, for only when we realise that we do indeed have choices can we can begin to choose. It is reassuring, then, to realise that people who are gullible to negative advice and images are also open to positive suggestion. I encourage patients to look at AIDS as a hurdle rather than the end of the line. I explain that my aim is to work with them to achieve their optimum health. Now this may take time, many months or years and, of course, nobody should be under any illusion about the amount of effort and persistence required. Unfortunately, many patients do not persevere, but there are others, however, who will accept the challenge.

Another important aspect concerns the will and its positive channeling. In any so-called 'terminal' disease, patients are often encouraged, albeit unintentionally, to take a passive stance. I believe that if there is not a definite commitment to be well then patients leave themselves open to all the social negative programming which starts with the HIV+ diagnosis. The fact is that attitude affects health and taking control of one's life is perhaps the first step to better health. This is why I place such an emphasis on making choices and decisions that suit the patient. Of course, if the patient decides imminent death is the likely outcome, then they will also attract the kind of people and situations which supports *this* view.

Some patients are so afraid of the HIV virus that even if they feel well they may still believe they are ill. I have noticed many patients continue to invest a great deal of power in the virus even when they are improving dramatically as a result of homœopathic treatment. By noticing such attitudes and bringing them to the attention of our patients we can perhaps help them to adjust their attitudes in a positive way.

Some people feel that it is better not to 'raise patient's hopes' by encouraging too positive an attitude. In some cases 'fighting spirit' is erroneously confused with denial. I prefer to encourage patients to keep an open mind, especially considering all the mis-information which exists, and to 'go for it', to *find out* what is achievable for themselves.

Evidently AIDS can be a catalyst for positive change, both for those directly affected as well as friends, family and even their homœopaths. For some patients it may be that AIDS leads to a reassessment of their lives, allowing them to be happier and to develop in all kinds of rich and previously unimagined ways. It is a curious fact that those with a strong syphilitic taint are often the most creative: Beethoven died from liver cirrhosis and was suicidal for much of his life; Van Gogh, of course, cut off his own ear in a uniquely syphilitic gesture while Schubert died from syphilis itself. I have known patients say that AIDS was the best thing that could have happened even where their lives have been shortened. AIDS can focus the mind on what is truly important in life. Every moment will be lived as if it were the last and the potential for love and forgiveness is huge. Sometimes people even find their true mission at this time which can heal them and allow them to live for many more years, as happened, for example, in the case of Edward Bach[10] who had cancer and went on to develop the famous flower remedies.

It may be that when seemingly well indicated remedies are not working, the patient's will to become healthy has been distorted at some deep level. This is at the level of belief structures and these may need uncovering before a person can move on in their life. For example, a patient may have been badly traumatised in their early life or even before birth which may block progress. Other therapies may come in useful here - rebirthing, cranial osteopathy, regression, psychotherapy, to name a few. Visualisation exercises and affirmations may be useful for patients with low self-belief.

We have to find where a person's true intention lies. Some patients become ill following a specific event such as the death of a partner, and, in some ways, this kind of case is simpler - the indicated remedy releases the blocked energy so they can move on. Others have had long-standing traumas going deep into the very fabric of their life. This type of person often arrives with mixed intentions; they would like to end their suffering but they find it difficult to feel a will to live (cf. Syphilitic miasm). They often have very deeply engrained fear. It is important to realise this otherwise we can feel frustrated when certain patients do not improve as we would wish. Sometimes homœopathic treatment will uncover the deep fear or belief structure and this may present unforeseen problems for the patient, and an unexpected reaction for the practitioner to handle. To take an example, imagine a patient whose energy has been suppressed because of an issue around their strong sexual drive; as soon as the patient is 'de-suppressed' the sexual drive will re-appear.

The tendency is for society either to revile people with AIDS or to pity them, neither attitude, in my opinion, being at all helpful. I like to establish a good practical working relationship with my patients, which means being frank in the advice that I give. If I perceive a patient is wasting my time and theirs, for example, if a patient sabotages their treatment carelessly through the taking of recreational drugs, I feel it is important to confront them on the issue. I insist that patients discontinue (gradually if necessary) any recreational drugs they are currently taking due to the effect on the action of remedies. Also, where treatments are paid for by a charity or other body, some patients may, in my opinion, abuse the system in a number of ways, such as not arriving for appointments or not taking the treatment seriously.

I have seen how being actively involved in making changes in lifestyle can be a valuable part of the patient's process of regaining health. I remember one man who pleaded to be allowed to continue taking his dope. He agreed, reluctantly, to stop smoking the drug for a few months and was thrilled with the effects of the homœopathic treatment; but almost as importantly he was delighted with himself for giving up smoking.

In my experience patients do not respond well to being treated like valuable china. In this respect there is a fine line to be drawn between sensitivity and mawkishness. From my perspective, it seems an important part of the healing relationship to treat the patient as a normal living human being with a blueprint for perfect health. I have also noticed that a sense of humour goes a long way!

It is important to maintain your energy when treating 'heavy' cases. Here is an exercise you may like to try when treating people with so-called 'terminal' diseases or low energy states where your own energy is likely to become depleted, it will help you feel more powerful and centred:

Sit in your chair in the consulting room. Be aware of the feelings of your physical body. Especially, be aware of the sensation of the contact between you and the chair. Feel the weight of your body, feel comfortable. Breathe slowly, regularly and deeply (without hyper-ventilating). Imagine drawing your breath up from your feet, through your legs, pelvic region, torso and into your head and then back down again so there is a flow of energy through your body. Enjoy this sensation. Now focus your attention on your pelvic region and imagine the energy being concentrated there and radiating outwards. Do the same for your heart centre and the 'third eye'. Now, in one split second be aware of all three centres with their concentrated and radiating energy. Send this energy in the direction of your patient, knowing that you will be 'refilled' at the same rate.

Flower essences are useful for the practitioner to avoid being overwhelmed by 'heavy' cases. For example I will often keep a glass of water with Bach Rescue Remedy on my desk. Alternatively try a combination of Bach Walnut, Crab Apple and Centaury which helps protect against negative influences. This combination can also be used in a mister and sprayed in the consultation room.

Psychological Issues

Although a lot has been written on this subject it warrants further examination.

AIDS is the ultimate twentieth century disease, surpassing even cancer in the fear it inspires. It is associated with powerlessness, despair and inevitable and imminent death. One spiritually aware patient with AIDS once told me that AIDS is about "hopelessness - not just hopelessness but hopelessness *beyond* hopelessness. A sort of damnation".

If we look at some of the words and images associated with AIDS we can vividly see some of the problems such patients face:

Victim ... hopelessness ... killer virus ... gay plague ... helplessness ... guilt ... divine vengeance ... isolation...fear... shame... desperation... death.

These words and images assault them from every corner of society: the media, the government, the health services, and their own family and friends.

The results of a positive HIV test may be very powerful: it is equated with death, doom and gloom. The practioner will have to give his support as well as remedies prescribed on the basis of the presenting emotional symptoms. Quite often the 'diagnosis' is a catalyst in that old or underlying problems are brought to the surface. This may, of course, be a great time of healing.

Useful remedies to bear in mind during this time include: *Aconite, Ignatia, Arsenicum, Phosphoric Acid, Aurum, the Calcium salts, Ambra Grisea, Argentum Nitricum, Carcinosin* and *Syphilinum* prescribed either singly or in combination.

The diagnosis of *any* 'terminal' disease (e.g. cancer) can have a powerful adverse effect on someone's overall level of health. In HIV disease there is not only fear of death and impending disability to contend with but also issues of guilt and stigmatisation.

Some families, despite their good intentions, may become maintaining factors in the patient's illness. Members of these families may have an inner need to be 'carers' and may resist, albeit subconsciously, any positive change in the patient's condition.

Many patients become confused at all the information and warnings they are proffered. Those who resist the conventional approach are often told that they are 'in denial'. There are many well-meaning health care professionals who are convinced that HIV is a certain killer. People who resist taking drug prophylaxis for PCP may be told that there is a high probability of developing the disease. These negative suggestions, albeit well meant, can be destructive to somebody in a vulnerable and suggestible state.

Many patients surround themselves with disease, death and dying and may, in their own minds, feel like a class apart (cf. *Hura Braziliensis*). For some people there may be a certain romance attached to AIDS. For example, after a funeral for one of his friends I heard one man sigh wistfully, "I'll be joining you soon". From a homœopathic perspective perhaps it is the tubercular miasm which is responsible for such morbid romanticism. Although remedies may help, the basic intent to live or die can be deeply entrenched.

Another interesting perspective came to light when I asked a patient who had responded well to treatment, "How would you feel if I offered you a tablet that would completely cure HIV and AIDS?" He paused for some while before admitting that he was unsure whether he would take my tablet because to do so would mean changing his whole life - getting a job, giving up his welfare benefits etc. People have even claimed falsely to be HIV+ in order to obtain social security benefits or services. So, some patients may be attached to a particular disease label and acknowledging this can bring about positive awareness together with the possibility of change.

There are people who have had 'fully blown AIDS' who survive for many years. Dr George F. Solomon who has carried out research into how the mind and emotions affects the immune system found that these survivors share the following characteristics: [11]

- **They are realistic and accept the AIDS diagnosis but do not take it as a death sentence.**

- **They have a fighting spirit and refuse to be 'helpless-hopeless'.**

- **They have changed lifestyles.**

- **They are assertive and have the ability to get out of stressful and unproductive situations.**

- **They are tuned into their own psychological and physical needs, and they take care of them.**

- **They are able to talk openly about their illness.**

- **They have a sense of personal responsibility for their health, and they look at the treating physician as a collaborator.**

- **They are altruistically involved with other persons with AIDS.**

Psychological Issues Around HIV/AIDS [12]

Shock
- of diagnosis and possible death
- over loss of hopes for good news

(*Aconite, Ignatia, Proteus, Argentum Nitricum, Carcinosin, Arsenicum, Calcarea Arsenicosum, Stramonium*)

Fear and anxiety
- uncertain prognosis and course of illness
- of disfigurement and disability
- effects of medication and treatment
- of isolation, abandonment and social/sexual rejection
- of infecting others and being infected by them
- of lover's ability to cope and his or her possible illness
- of loss of cognitive, physical, social and work abilities

(*Phosphorus, Arsenicum, Calcarea Carbonica, Dys. Co. Calcarea Sulphurica, Syphilinum*)

Depression
- over "inevitability" of physical decline
- over absence of a cure
- over the virus controlling future life
- over limits imposed by ill health, and possible social, occupational, emotional and sexual rejection
- from self blame and recrimination for being vulnerable to infection in the first place.

(*Aurum, Carcinosin, Phosphoric Acid, Mercurius, Syphilinum*)

Psychological Issues Around HIV/AIDS (cont)

Anger and frustration
- over inability to overcome the virus
- over new and involuntary health/lifestyle restrictions
- at being 'caught out' and the uncertainty of the future

(Proteus, Anacardium, Syphilinum, Nux Vomica)

Guilt
- over past 'misdemeanours' resulting in illness self 'punishment'
- over possibly having spread infection to others
- over being homosexual or a drug user

(Thuja, Carcinosin, Bromium, Calcarea Bromatum, Arsenicum, Syphilinum, Mercurius)

Obsessive disorders
- relentless searching for new diagnostic evidence on body; faddism over health and diets
- preoccupation with death and decline, and avoidance of new infections

(Arsenicum, Syphilinum)

The Healing Power Within

The following is based on a sheet I give to all patients of mine who have tested HIV+.

Whenever we choose to receive a therapy such as homœopathy we are also connecting to a new way of looking at our health, our lives and the meaning of disease. Western medicine takes a mechanical view of our bodies; a bit like with a car, when something goes wrong we change the oil or remove an offending cog, etc. It also tends to put all the blame for any 'malfunction' outside of ourselves. The best example of this is the idea of bacteria and viruses. It cannot be denied that these exist, but what we have to ask is whether they actually *cause* the disease.

The bacteria or virus is there, the disease is there, but does one cause the other? Some holistic practitioners believe not. If you have flies around your dustbin do the flies *cause* the dustbin?[13] Obviously not. This may all sound academic and perhaps irrelevant, but it has great consequences when we try to treat the disease. If we believe that bacteria and viruses are the sole cause of disease then the natural step is to want to kill them. It sounds logical and this is where antibiotics come in.

Antibiotics were the great medical discovery of this century and, in one sense, they are an amazing piece of medical technology. But several decades later we are faced with problems. In a sense, antibiotics were designed to do the work of the immune system, but their overuse has led to a situation where bacteria are becoming resistant to the old antibiotics. New and more powerful drugs take their place (which cause their own problems within the body) and the bacteria become resistant to these as well. Added to this, antibiotics themselves are immuno-suppressant (one of the results of this is the emergence of Candida, or thrush, which is now being recognised as a major problem). Even Alexander Fleming, the inventor of antibiotics, himself saw and warned against the abuse of these drugs as early as 1942. Some would argue that the abuse of antibiotics may be implicated in immune system problems like AIDS.

Therapies such as homœopathy and acupuncture attempt to treat people as whole, intelligent beings. They assume the presence within and around the body of a guiding, controlling energy which, in ancient Chinese Medicine, is called *Chi*, in India, *Prana*, and in the Western tradition is known as the *Vital Force*. What is this energy, then? We all know what it is but many of us have difficulty remembering the experience! It has several functions: it is creative - it can make new tissue and so ensures growth; it can heal or repair damaged tissue; it maintains the integrity of the body - for example by repelling or killing invading organisms. Generally it allows for our survival.

This Vital Force is intelligent and works in a meaningful way. What we call disease is, in fact, the Vital Force's way of expressing disorder. Symptoms, then, can be likened to the oil light coming on in our car telling us that something is wrong. But in order to cure the problem we must go to the cause. It would be no good, to continue our car analogy, just ripping out the oil light. If we did that the engine would inevitably fail.

One of the problems we have in the West is we always want instant results. Life seems to get faster and faster and we want everything yesterday, if possible! It is the same in medicine. We want a drug which will take away our pains, our skin problems, our sufferings right now. One result of this is that we forget that the body will often heal itself if we give just it a chance and the other result is we ply ourselves with powerful drugs which can make the problem worse.

Homœopaths have noticed that if a problem on, say, the skin, is made to disappear by cortisone cream, for example, another problem takes its place - perhaps asthma. This is because the *whole* person has not been taken into account, but only one part. The Vital Force was just doing its job telling us there was a problem by sending out symptoms onto the skin and we take those symptoms away, but the root of the problem has not been cured. So the Vital Force has to find another expression for the problem - thus we get asthma.

What happens when we start becoming healthier, for example during homœopathic treatment, is that symptoms on the skin and the extremities *may* temporarily get worse while our general state improves. We may feel more energy, less anxious, better able to deal with the stresses in life but, for example, we develop a rash. This is a good sign. And this is why it is so important to keep in touch with your practitioner during treatment and *not* rush out to buy something from the chemist which may undo all the good work that has been done.

Homœopathy (and other holistic therapies) aims to put your health on an altogether better level, rather than just curing symptoms. But this may take time, so do *persevere* with the treatment. Working with your homœopath regularly over a period of time (weeks, months or even years) can be very satisfying as you watch your general health improve. On the other hand expecting a miracle (although these *do* occur from time to time) in one or two sessions is not fair on you or your practitioner. Remember, it took all these years to get where you are now so it may take time to work through the problems.

Always ask your practitioner any questions if you feel unsure about the treatment. Remember, this is *your* health and life. Take control and be interested in it. *This* is the first step to better health.

What Causes Immunodeficiency?

Much effort has been expended trying to find a single
cause of HIV/AIDS but it seems more likely to be a
combination of factors which confers susceptibility on
some people. Alan Jones reports:

> "The orthodox approach is based upon cellular
> pathology i.e. only the virus & its effect on the physical
> body is considered. The wholistic concept is concerned
> with the broader effects on the physical, etheric and
> astral components of the human being and if we apply
> some lateral thinking to these symptom pictures, it seems
> obvious that they result from secondary influences and,
> indeed, that HIV and AIDS could themselves be
> secondary to some more profound condition."

Dr G Orth reported in 'Raum und Zeit' 56/92:

> "I have been able to establish that in every case (of HIV
> or AIDS) that has come to my attention, the patient had
> already been immune suppressed by drugs or by
> antibiotics or some other heavy immune suppressants.
> Every medicine that is used in AIDS is immune
> suppressant. The mucous membranes, these highly
> antiseptic entry points to the human body, are further
> perforated and eroded."

The following factors may, in my experience, lead to a compromised immune system and therefore greater susceptibility to AIDS. One may presume that with greater presentation of the following in any individual case, the more likely is there to be problems with immunity.

Family heredity. The miasmatic background is usually strongly active and complex in AIDS cases: a typical family background of a patient may include cancer, tuberculosis, diabetes and schizophrenia.

Personal medical history is typically poor, with quantities of antibiotics and other suppressive drug treatments throughout life.

Vaccinations may also have been frequently received, especially those for foreign travel such as yellow fever and typhoid. It is useful to enquire specifically about the vaccination history and any reactions that may have occurred.

Venereal diseases, often repeated, are also common in the medical history. One man I treated who used to be a prostitute had contracted gonorrhœa 50 times. Three to four bouts of gonorrhœa is quite common, together with one or more incidents of syphilis.

Recreational drug abuse: many people with AIDS have a history of a great deal of drug abuse and have often experimented with many different drugs. However, I believe injected heroin to be the most damaging.

Poor living conditions and/or diet: e.g. homelessness.

Trauma, emotional or physical, such as torture, beatings, murder of close relatives, sexual abuse, grief, much love disappointment.

Candidiasis

Candida is a common, often seemingly intractable, problem in HIV/AIDS. Candida albicans is a normal inhabitant of the lower bowel and it is usually kept under control by the high pH values which are maintained by lactobacilli, another of the bowel's inhabitants. Antibiotics are one class of drug which can upset the balance of the bowel flora by killing lactobacilli. This then allows the entry of other morbific bacteria thus reducing the pH value and providing the right conditions for the proliferation of yeasts, moulds and viruses, the most common of which is Candida albicans which can spread throughout the gastro-intestinal tract.

Could then Candida albicans be one of the 'lynch pins' in the successful treatment of the HIV/AIDS syndrome or is it merely one more scavenger of an already ravaged immune system? It has certainly been my experience that standard homœopathy can achieve a great deal but is frequently hindered by proliferation of Candida within the system.

The following is reproduced by kind permission of Australian homœopath Alan Jones from an unpublished paper:

Dr Orion Truss from Alabama, USA was the first to recognise the symptom picture of candidiasis and demonstrated that the spores of intestinal candida could enter the blood stream and cause 'partial paralysis of the immune system'.

Many orthodox practitioners have steadfastly refused to accept the reality of systemic candidiasis, since the yeast is not detected in stool samples in much greater quantities than normal, except when the patient is extremely sick. Cross infection of the colon does occur, however, particularly when the pH drops, when the candida myceliates and the spores penetrate the mucosal walls instead of passing into the lower bowel.

Truss established a research centre funded by a grateful patient, and developed a biochemical/pathological model which explained the ætiology of systemic candidiasis. Of particular interest was his finding that red blood cells, which are normally elastic enough to pass through 'sieves' with a diameter one third that of the blood cell, lost that elasticity in the presence of Candida. He also noticed a distinct reduction in available potassium & phosphorus in blood infected with Candida. The combined effect of these is to restrict blood supply, particularly oxygen and nutrients, to vital organs with fine capilliaries such as the brain.

Truss recognised the symptoms of emotional instability, poor concentration, defective memory, vertigo, headaches and depression as being directly related to brain function, and referred to them as 'brain symptoms' as opposed to mental or 'neurotic symptoms'. The most common symptom picture of systemic candidiasis includes:

Mind	*Concentration; Difficult*
	Memory; Weakness Of
	Confidence. Loss Of; Self, In, In Hysteria
Head	*Vertigo*
Mouth	*Aphthae*
	Ulcers
Stomach	*Desires; Sugar*
Abdomen	*Distension; Gas, By; Menses, Before*
	Eating, After
	Flatulence
	Hypochondria; Pain; Right Side
	Pain; Flatulent Colic; Hypogastrium
	Duodenum; Catarrhal Inflammation; Gurgling
	Liver; Congestion
Female	*Vagina; Itching*
	Leucorrhea

*More than 90% of immunosuppressed patients respond
favourably to the candida treatment. Those that do not have
usually failed to follow the strict sugar-free diet which
accompanies the treatment.*

*Patients return after 2-3 weeks for a second consultation with a
marked improvement in emotional and physical well-being, and
almost complete loss of sugar craving. Overall, they 'feel better
in themselves', more stable emotionally, with an increased energy
level, improved appetite without bloating, and often a reduction
in weight.*

*Use of the Candida Albicans nosode seems to be obligatory for a
successful resolution. Early attempts with well-indicated
constitutional remedies gave little success. The first nosodes were
prepared by hand succussion of the lysated ferment, prepared
for an earlier proving, to a 30C potency using the Korsakoff
method. This proved remarkably successful when prescribed
daily for 10 days, but often aggravated. Patients were restricted
to a strict sugar and yeast free diet. Some aggravations followed
breaking this diet, but others deteriorated nevertheless.
Progressively higher potencies of 1M, 5M, 10M etc. were used
until there were no reports of aggravation, which was achieved
at the 20M potency.*

*A liver-stimulating remedy, usually in the 30C potency three
times daily before meals, was added to the prescription with even
better results, particularly in the reduction of bloating, nausea
and energy level. Chelidonium used as a drainage remedy in 3X
potency was used initially with good results, but Lycopodium 30
has proved consistently better.*

*Although these results were very encouraging, the incidence of
relapse of symptoms, particularly after drinking wine or eating
sugar-rich foods raised the holistic approach of treating the
etheric and astral bodies. Subsequent treatment using 50M and
CM potencies of Candida nosode supported by higher potencies
of liver remedies was introduced, with marked improvement in
the long term success rate.*

Where symptoms included vaginitis, oral thrush or cystitis, these were markedly improved by Nystatin 3X, although it had little effect on the chronic symptoms and none on the mental.

Penicillin & Erythromycin in potency had no effect but Cortisone 10M gave a marked improvement in the totality of symptoms.

Sepia, Folliculinum & Oestrogen, used to stimulate oestrogen production, gave no relief to the gynæcological symptoms from which it was deduced that the interference from candida was not with the production of ovarian hormones but with the lack of response to them, which was verified by blood and urine tests. Indeed hormone stimulation may aggravate because of its effect on the thyroid, adrenals and pituitary through a negative feedback mechanism.

Thyreostimuline 3X and Carbo Vegetabilis 6 improved energy levels & digestion problems, and were used frequently in early trials. Mandragora 3X & Serotonin 6X were of great assistance in some cases.

Lycopodium proved invaluable in most cases, and became the supporting remedy of choice in later trials. However, in the early trials it frequently aggravated the mentals and was particularly sensitive to sugars. Later a further distinct correlation between the aggravations and the use of the birth control pill was apparent. After some experimentation the 30, 200 & 1M potencies, prescribed 3 times daily before meals, were found to be most effective.

Supplements:
Lactobacillus Acidophilus tablets, because of their potential to recolonise the intestinal tract with desirable bacteria should have proved advantageous, but invariably caused a deterioration in condition in the early stages of treatment. The 500 mgm tablets, taken twice daily for 2 weeks, were useful after completion of the homœopathic treatment particularly if the patient took further antibiotics.
Vitamin B Complex and Vitamin C proved useful at all times.

Dietary Restrictions:
Overly strict diets are often counterproductive. Although
avoiding obvious allergic reactions, the diets often prescribed
for candida patients are so restrictive as to result in poor
nutritional uptake, which is hardly conducive to improving
immune function. However, sugar must be avoided absolutely,
and the following restrictions have proved adequate:

100% avoidance:
All forms of sugar, including glucose, fructose, honey, soft fruits,
fruit juices, dried fruit, sweets, cakes, biscuits, jams, marmalade,
refined carbohydrates, soft drinks. Alcohol, particularly beer &
wine, vegemite (marmite), mushrooms, canned foods.
Antibiotics, cortisones, birth control pills.

Partial avoidance:
Fried foods, fats, colourings, hard cheeses, smoked meats,
vegetable juices.

From the evidence presented by Alan Jones, assuming that
candida is another miasm, it would seem likely that
nosodes prepared from other opportunistic organisms may
be extremely useful in tackling AIDS. (See section on
Nosodes).

Other remedies which may prove useful in more localised
conditions (e.g. oro-pharynx) include: *Natrum Phosphoricum,*
Kali Muriaticum, Borax.

There are additional naturopathic methods of candida
control which have been found to be useful:

Caprystatin
(also known as caprylic acid and available as Mycopryl)
This is an anti-fungal fatty acid, extracted from coconut,
which mimics the fatty acids produced by normal bowel
flora. Caprystatin is preferable to the anti-fungal drug
Nystatin, because the latter is itself yeast based, which
ultimately results in more colonies of yeast developing

after the drug is stopped. Caprylic acid on the other hand has no such rebound effect when its use ceases and has the additional benefit of allowing the re-colonisation of the gut with friendly bacteria.

The following herbal medications, are worth experimenting with either singly or in combination:

Aloe Vera
Has an anti-fungal action. Also improves the local acidity balance.
Dosage: 1-2 teaspoonfuls in water, twice daily.

Tea Tree Oil
For external use only. Powerful anti-fungal agent. Useful for localised fungal infections of the skin.

Taheebo
Useful in catarrhal problems caused by candida. Take as a tea substitute.

Berberine containing herbs
These include Berberis Vulgaris, Berberis Aquifolium and Hydrastis Canadensis. Berberine is useful for preventing candida after antibiotic use, and also encourages friendly bacteria. It is an anti-diarrhoea agent when there is chronic bowel infection. It has a reputation for destroying bacteria, yeasts, viruses and cancer cells.
Dosage: 1 - $1^1/_2$ teaspoons of tincture (dilute 1:5) of any of the above plants, three times daily.

Other anti-candida approaches include:

Lactobacillus Acidophilus and **Bifidobacteria** (preferably in yoghourt).
Garlic capsules which have a general 'anti-biotic' effect.
Oleic acid (as virgin, first pressing olive oil).

54

Materia Medica

AGNUS CASTUS

This remedy seems peculiarly suited to the AIDS condition (one of two remedies listed under the rubric 'AIDS' in the Complete Repertory). Its main keynote is loss of sexual power and impotence (usually in men), a picture of sexual excess. This is usually accompanied by depression, discouragement and dissatisfaction. There may be a fear of death through AIDS. The patient may have been extra-ordinarily active, sexually, at one time (some gay men claimed to have had 1000 sexual partners in one year) but now the sex drive has disappeared and has left depression, apathy and weakness.

He finds it difficult to sustain an erection. Life only seems worth living when the sexual drive is high. Thus we see the term 'jaded rakes' in our materia medicas which expresses this feeling of spent force or impotence (on all levels). The patient may also feel frustrated and irritable with himself at his loss of power. Another major pointer in this remedy's picture is a history of repeated gonorrhoea which is so common amongst people with AIDS. There may also be prostate problems. The patient looks older than his years, premature old age. To prescribe this remedy, it will be necessary to delve into the sexual history of the patient, the degree of promiscuity and number of gonorrhoea episodes.

(Related to *Picric Acid, Selenium, Phosphoric Acid, China, Lycopodium*)

AIDS NOSODE

The *AIDS nosode* derives from several different sources which have either been proved or used intuitively. One of these, a blood sample from a man who later died of AIDS, was prepared by Ainsworths pharmacy in London and has been given a meditative proving (i.e. not ingested) by Misha Norland and a group of homoeopathy students. The main themes they uncovered included a sense of lack of boundaries or vulnerability, the feeling of having done something so terrible that they cannot even talk about it; this is coupled with a feeling of deep isolation and alienation. One prover who had experienced sexual abuse earlier in her life had a poignant healing reaction to the remedy.

I am grateful to Marc Blausten and Shereen Joshua, homœopaths practising in Birmingham for their clinical observations and intuitive information about the *AIDS nosode* as prepared radionically. The following is based on notes regarding an *AIDS nosode* prepared radionically on a digital machine made by Bill McGurk[14]. For those with such a machine the rate used is: **98 (10) 5861.** The information is partly obtained through clinical feedback from a number of (non-HIV+) cases and partly through intuitive deduction. This information is included as material for further research and is not intended to be definitive. The author would be glad to hear of any reader's experiences with the remedy.

Lack Of Responsibility
People live for today and to hell with the consequences. They don't care. Refuse to take responsibility.

Blame
People blame others or their situation for their suffering (for example, they blame the practitioner or the remedies).
Blame is interesting. We are 100% responsible for our lives; we create and change. Blaming is attempting to put responsibilty onto someone else; which means blaming is disempowering oneself.

Denial Of Knowledge Of Right And Wrong
Therefore there is no need to be personally responsible for their actions.
'If you can get away with it, why not?'
Complete loss of spiritual dimension or perspective leading to disrespectful, dangerous attitude to self and others. No heed of Law of Karma.

Very Fearful
The disease inspires fear, because it is not understood. Lots of scare mongering. People think they can become a victim of it, that they have no control over their destiny. Fear = No Control. Fear destroys the immune system.

Victim Mentality
They become fearful of the very things they are not taking responsibility for, e.g. fear of being poor, but they do nothing in life to change it. Just blame others for their plight. Stuck in it.

Agoraphobia
Fearful of life.

Greedy
Greed is based on a fear of not having enough which is a result of a fear of poverty. Which in turn creates poverty as the Earth's resources are depleted.

Demanding
Want and expect instant results in their lives, want instant gratification.

Insistent
People who want a quick fix to get back to normal.
(Which was what caused the problem in the first place-
but they didn't want to change).

Work
Has to be faster. Life has to be faster. Get there before
the next person.

Play
Children want something and they get it. (They watch
television consistently, continually occupied: computers,
fast computer games, stimulate, stimulate.) So they
become solitary, introverted, bored. Lack the social
skills. Children are spoilt. If they don't get what they
want they have tantrums (children *and* adults). Many
children need the AIDS nosode.

Food
Fast food, processed. Microwaves. No time to cook. Life
is too busy. Children want sweets now, sugar addicts.

Sex
Early promiscuity. Promiscuity generally. Miasms can be
communicated through sex. Very open energy fields may
communicate miasms. Blood transfusions. Lots of
partners = lots of miasms.

Overindulgence
in anything beyond what is enjoyable. Desire for
constant stimulation. everyone lives life in the fast lane.
Constant barrage of sensory input, which is another
good way of avoiding ourselves. Put a huge strain on
nervous and immune systems.

Anger
When any of the above is pointed out they are forced out
of denial to look at themselves. But they may choose to
remain sick.

Materialistic

There has never been so much available to so many.
People are fulfilling their dreams of material success but
it is not enough. People are searching for security. True
security is never attained in the physical world alone.
They are left feeling unfulfilled and disappointed, as they
have material wealth but are not satisfied.

Delusion-Time

Time is speeding up, or at least a sense of. The paradox
is the more you do the faster time goes.

Physical Symptoms

• Weakness, constantly run down.
• Lymphatics are affected e.g. constant tonsillitis,
appendicitis
• Children get chronic glandular swellings, constant
colds, anything lymphatic.

General

The disease (AIDS) is centred in the Sacral centre - the
centre of physical desire and sex organs. Desires are out
of control. Also, physiologically speaking it is the seat of
the immune system (the reservoir of *Chi* is here).
The *AIDS nosode* is very good for M.E. type states.
People who need this remedy are often not willing to
change their lifestyle. They adamantly refuse to accept
that it has anything to do with their disease.
After the remedy, a great deal may come to the surface,
which has to happen for people to heal themselves.
With regards to potency, it is the same as any remedy.

AMBRA GRISEA

I believe this is an under used remedy. It is indicated in states that come on after repeated grief or shocks (people with lots of friends who have died of AIDS) It is one step further on from *Ignatia*. The state of shock has turned into one of confusion or emotional breakdown. They feel really ungrounded. There is a sense of escaping from reality, of dreaminess (although this may not be obvious; some quite apparently tough types need this remedy). Lots of worries. They think about their emotions a lot which takes them 'up into their head'. Trembling. All kinds of strange symptoms that don't seem to add up (cf. *Ignatia's* hysteria). Tired and worn out from too much emotion and worry. Faded look. Itching with no eruption. In the Materia Medicas we read that *Ambra Grisea* is worse for embarrassment. We can see this in the broader sense of being mentally overwhelmed.

Ambra Grisea worked very well in the case of a forty-four year old man who was worn out, sweating profusely, and trembling. Several of his friends had died within a short space of time. Although *Mercurius* seemed indicated it was *Ambra Grisea* which helped. Cf: *Cocculus, Carcinosin,* and *Ignatia.*

ANTHRACINUM

I have used this remedy successfully in cases of whitlow with red streaks running up the arm, but it is worth considering where there is exhaustion and collapse accompanied by burning pains and malignancy. In this respect it is similar to *Arsenicum* and *Tarentula Cubensis* but to an even more intense degree. There may frequently be boils (cf. *Echinacea*), carbuncles, ulceration, foul secretions (cf. *Pyrogen*), swellings which may be blue/black, septic fever, gangrene. The picture is one of septicaemia.

ARSENICUM ALBUM

Little need be said about this polychrest. The anxiety
experienced is insidious, as if it is eating away at the
patient. When people look as if they are dying they usually
need *Arsenicum* or *Carbo Vegetabilis.* Tremendous weakness
with fear of dying. Very chilly. Sometimes patients who
need this remedy may say that they are not anxious. One
women said she trusted God to save her but she was
clearly terrified. The patient may say they feel lost and
plead with you to help. 'You have got to help me', one man
said over and over. In both cases *Arsenicum* worked
wonderfully. In the right cases it can almost literally bring
people back from the dead. Also consider the related
remedies *China Arsenicosum* and *Calcarea Arsenicosum.*

AZT

Also known as Azidothymidine or Zidovudine, this anti-viral
drug which is one of the main tools of the medical
approach, can cause nausea, vomiting, insomnia, wasting,
anaemia and leucopenia/neutropenia in many patients. It is
definitely useful, in potency, for treating the side effects of
this drug (and perhaps other chemotherapy drugs), but
does not seem to positively influence T4 cell counts.

THE CALCIUM SALTS

The *Calcarea* salts are probably the most useful remedies in the Materia Medica for AIDS and AIDS-related disease. They are listed for third stage syphilis in the Repertory. People who need the calcium salts tend in general to be vulnerable. Imagine a new-born baby who needs total protection - *Calcarea Carbonica* is often indicated in infants - or the calcareous shell of a crab protecting the soft tissues underneath. This is the essence of the potentised calcium salts. In AIDS there is a lack of boundaries; anything can enter the system and establish itself - bacteria, viruses, protozoans, fungi. So naturally the patient feels - and is - vulnerable. (If we look at the depletion of the ozone layer, which has come at about the same time as AIDS, we see this same vulnerability mirrored on a planetary scale).
This is compounded by the 'us and them' aspect of AIDS. So there is a great deal of fear which leads to protection and withdrawal (see *Homœopathy and Minerals*).[15] On the physical level, the calcium salts cover the symptoms of respiratory problems, brain abscesses, diarrhoea, night sweats - a considerable span of the common AIDS - related symptoms.

CALCAREA CARBONICA

Perhaps best summed up by the delusions, 'About to sink into annihilation', and 'Body being dashed to pieces'. There may be a feeling that their world, indeed their body, is disintegrating, together with a fear of death. If you ask why they fear death they may say it is a fear of not existing. (*Arsenicum*, for example, has a fear of losing control).

Scholten describes how the *Calcareas* fear what others think of them, and this often correlates with how patients who are HIV+ feel towards the rest of society. With *Calcarea Carbonica* there may be a paucity of symptoms but with a feeling that the state affects the patient's very structure. With calcium being such a major part of our physical structure this is not surprising.

Calcarea Carbonica is useful in all kinds of respiratory diseases. One man had a definite shadow on his lung and was suspected of having PCP, and this was cured by *Calcarea Carbonica*. The *Calcarea* picture also includes chronic debilitating diarrhœa.

Calcarea Carbonica is frequently perceived as a remedy for people who are bulky and flabby in their build, but I have given it to some quite skinny people. Some of them have lost weight through a debilitating illness. But the head seems quite large relative to the body (like the physical proportions of a baby), and the head is sweaty.

I have found that under an acute *Mercurius* picture there often lurks a *Calcarea* constitutional state. The fearful state can also sometimes mislead one into prescribing *Phosphorus*.

CALC BROMATUM

A case will demonstrate the main strands of this remedy:

Case: The patient is a thirty-two year old woman who is HIV+. She has a history of alcoholism and drug abuse, more specifically heroin. She is also taking anti-depressants, and sleeping pills. The drug abuse started thirteen years ago after she gave away her baby because she could not cope. Having retaken charge of the baby after a change of mind it was then taken away from her again by the authorities because it was felt to be in the child's best interests. Since then, she felt, her life was a long slippery downwards slope.

She feels much guilt, depression and she continues to think a great deal about the baby. She has marked mood swings, violent dreams and she is absent minded. She goes to bed late because her mind is so alert. She also mentions a pressing pain at the back of her head which started after she was hit on the head with a hammer by her boyfriend!

I prescribed several remedies at various times (including *Medorrhinum., Mercurius, Syphilinum, X-ray*) which all helped but did not get to the root of the case.

The remedy which repertorised highest was *Calcarea Carbonica.* In my experience, however, *Calcarea Carbonica* doesn't have the degree of trauma and emotional turmoil as presented here. If not *Calcarea Carbonica* could it possibly be one of the other *Calcarea* salts? According to Jan Scholten the themes of *Calcarea Bromatum* are as follows:

Calcium	*Bromatum*
What do others think	Guilt
Sensitive to criticism	Restless, escape
Insecurity	Passion, instinct
Shyness	Psychotic
Fear	
Protection	
Withdrawal	

My patient looked like a typical *Calcarea* type, fair haired and slightly overweight. She had a love of the sea, feeling markedly better there (*Bromatum*). I could also see how she might fear that people would think her guilty for giving away her baby thirteen years ago (the main essence of *Calcarea Bromatum*). Boericke also mentions sleeplessness as a major symptom of this remedy.

Rx: *Calcarea Bromatum 30,* one a night for a week.

The response was dramatic. One week later she had
given up her sleeping pills and anti-depressants
entirely and cut her Valium down to half of the original
dosage. She started sleeping well with no unpleasant
dreams. Her moods stabilised. The period returned
normally (2 days after starting the remedy). She said
she felt like her old self.

Another use for *Calcarea Bromatum* is in gay men, where
there is much guilt about sexuality (cf. *Thuja, Natrum
Muriaticum, Carcinosin*). They have a fear of what others will
think. One man I treated had sleeplessness, a swollen
testicle together with tremendous guilt about sex. I gave
him *Calcarea Bromatum* and he became even more despairing
with guilt. He needed *Bromium*, which cured. The *Calcarea
Bromatum* exposed the undiluted guilty feelings which are
the essence of *Bromium*.

One function of the *Calcarea* component may be to
'uncover' that which lies beneath. I have observed this
effect in other cases where *Calcarea Carbonica* had been
prescribed, following which the patient became more
anxious.

In *Calcarea Bromatum* we see tremendous restlessness
with a desire to escape. This often means resorting to hard
or soft recreational drugs. This is definitely a syphilitic
remedy (the Complete Repertory mentions it under the
rubric 'Stage 3 Syphilis' and so can look like *Aurum* or
Mercurius). but interestingly , it can also look like a cross
between *Medorrhinum* (i.e. better by the sea) and
Syphilinum. There is a tendency to all kinds of brain disease
(I have prescribed it in a case of suspected brain tumour).
They may have all the typical *Calcarea Carbonica* cravings
and also crave chocolate.

CALCAREA ARSENICOSUM

Here was a remedy I knew very little about but, using Jan
Scholten's ideas, I prescribed it to a certain HIV+ patient
who works in a very high powered, stressful job. In some
ways he is quite *Arsenicum* but tries to hide his fears
because he doesn't want others to think he is falling apart.
He had also had recurring kidney problems, for which
Calcarea Arsenicosum is known. Because of the continuing
stress of his job I gave him a packet of *Calcarea Arsenicosum*
1M which he took whenever he felt the need. He called them
his 'anti-stress' pills and they worked very well.

One other patient, to whom I gave *Calcarea Arsenicosum,* had
been in shock following his HIV+ test result. He had a
tremendous fear of death and it seemed as if he might need
Arsenicum but his appearance (*Calcarea Carbonica*
stockiness) combined with a desire for soup (only 12
remedies listed of which *Calcarea Arsenicosum* is one)
suggested *Calcarea Arsenicosum* which definitely helped.

Boericke mentions chronic malaria in the *Calcarea
Arsenicosum* picture and, although I have not used it for this
condition, it is possible that it may be indicated for
anxious patients who have suffered much malaria in the
past. Indeed, many AIDS manifestations (for example,
intermittent inflammatory and febrile processes) fit Rajan
Sankaran's description of a malaria miasm in *'The Substance
of Homoeopathy'.* [16]

Especially, think of *Calcarea Arsenicosum* when the patient
looks like *Arsenicum* but where there is pathology centred
around the pancreas or kidneys.

CALCAREA PHOSPHORICA

One might expect this remedy to be frequently indicated in
AIDS patients, given the strong tubercular nature of the
condition. In the remedy picture, there is tremendous
restlessness and boredom, they cannot settle. They feel
they do not belong to any particular group or family, so
they wander from group to group, relationship to
relationship, with a constant sense of dissatisfaction. They
may adopt a wild lifestyle in order to assuage their
boredom. This craving for excitement is reflected in their
food desires - piquant, savoury and spicy foods. *Calcarea
Phosphorica* is of course strongly related to *Tuberculinum*,
the main difference being that *Calcarea Phosphorica* tends to
have more insecurity, especially about their learning
abilities or their ability to be part of a group. It is also a
remedy which can be useful for convalescence after long
debilitating illnesses.

CALCAREA SULPHURICA

I have found this to be a useful remedy in skin problems
especially where the patient feels insecure about his
attractiveness to others. One man I treated had appalling
psoriasis with cracking of the skin and extensive
desquamation all over the body. He was depressed
because he felt so unattractive. I began treating him with
Graphites and followed this up with *Calcarea Sulphurica.* In
two weeks he was amazed by the improvement. Because of
the sulphur component, *Calcarea Sulphurica* is also good for
skin complaints following extensive drugging, e.g.
antibiotics. There may also be acne, wounds or burns with
yellow discharge and swollen glands.

CARBO VEGETABILIS

Useful after long illness where a person is convalescing. Profound weakness. This may or may not be accompanied by the characteristic flatulence, abdominal distension and eructation. States following extensive drugging especially where it affects the digestive system. Sometimes worth alternating with *Nux Vomica* to help clear the picture. Can hardly think - very slow (unlike *China* which often has a very active mind). In the *Carbo Vegetabilis* state there is a sense as if the whole system has slowed down, everything has stagnated - the mind, the digestive system, the circulation. convalescence.

CARCINOSIN

Very often indicated for people with HIV/AIDS. Suppressed fear. Tremendous fear about anything. Fear may be controlled; not necessarily the obvious fear of *Phosphorus* or *Arsenicum*. This is natural when one considers the stigma surrounding HIV and AIDS. (cf. *Calcarea Arsenicosum* which has hidden fear but less combined mental and physical suppression). In patients who need *Carcinosin* one sees the fear coming through the eyes. History of traumas, shocks, grief, broken relationships, often one on top of another. Everything is suppressed - mentally and physically so that the energy is low. Vague all-pervading depression. Helplessness. Futility. Lack of self esteem. Life feels empty. May reject or desire sympathy. AIDS, like cancer, is a disease with a good deal of fear attached. Weakness from or after strong emotions. Crushed spirit. History of liver disease. Clears the way for other remedies. May be good to repeat remedy fairly frequently (e.g. 12c twice daily; or 10m, one as required).

Carcinosin may be combined sequentially with other nosodes e.g. *Carcinosin, Medorrhinum* and *Thuja*; or

Carcinosin, Tuberculinum, Thuja, or *Carcinosin, Tuberculinum, Syphilinum..* There may exist a clear TB miasm in the patient's history which has been overlaid with tremendous emotional suppression.

CHINA

Very sensitive, sometimes quite refined, delicate. Pale, washed out, not really in their body. Physically they are depleted but mentally they can be quite active. They are very much in their heads. Much theorising. A confirming symptom is many plans and ideas for the future but no energy to fulfil them, so they feel frustrated.[17] Whining. They feel unloved and abandoned, discouraged. (*China Boliviana* also has a strong, painful sense of humiliation) Can look like a combination of *Pulsatilla, Lycopodium*, and *Sulphur.* There is an unhappy restlessness. Delusion he is unfortunate, unhappy. Feels persecuted. Feels opposed and tormented by everybody.

Compared to *Carbo Vegetabilis, China's* abdominal wind tends to be more trapped. May not feel better from passing wind.

Many AIDS patients suffer from loss of vital fluids at some point, e.g. after profuse night sweats, chronic diarrhoea, vomiting or other acute illnesses. So it may be worth enquiring about this in the consultation. Useful remedy for diarrhoea after antibiotics. The patient is often very liverish. They may not want to move, although occupation may make them feel better mentally. Appetite may be poor until they start eating when the appetite will improve.

I have used it in combination with *Hydrastis* in 6x, after a person has lost much weight following illness. This may help to build them up and improve their appetite cf. *Alfalfa.*

COCCULUS

This remedy has confusion and disorientation even more
marked than that of *Ambra Grisea*. They really cannot think
properly and even feel physically dizzy with emotion.
Again, like *Ambra Grisea*, useful after multiple grief or
emotional trauma. Dazed sensation (similar to 'jet-lag'). I
used it in a case of ME/AIDS very successfully. The woman
had a history of emotional trauma, and felt tremendously
nauseous, exhausted, feverish. She looked quite fragile and
was very sensitive or allergic to all kinds of things. She was
very spaced out. *Cocculus* helped enormously. Another
case was a man who had experienced many deaths
amongst his friends. It was as if he had been hit by a car; he
was totally dazed and disorientated. I was tempted to
make a routine prescription of *Ignatia* in this case but
Cocculus was the remedy that was needed.

COFFEA

I recall an interesting case of a woman who looked like she
was dying. She was very thin, weak and frail and extremely
anxious. I prescribed *Arsenicum* and the following week
one would not have recognised her as the same person. She
came in cheerfully, looking strong and bright. She was
incredibly excited about her rapid improvement. A few
weeks later she came back with some strange symptoms
which did not seem to make sense: a persistent cough,
pains in her limbs and sleeplessness at night. Eventually I
realised that her excitement at becoming well had caused
symptoms in itself. She was suffering from 'ailments from
joy'. *Coffea* worked very quickly. Another patient was
receiving chemotherapy that had made him feel mentally
hyperactive and unable to sleep; again *Coffea* helped.

CYCLOSPORIN

This is an extract of a fungus used allopathically to suppress immune function in organ-transplanted patients. It may be of use therefore in stimulating the immune system in immuno-compromised patients when used homœopathically. Clinical experience seems to indicate that it is slow acting and gives variable results but may increase T4 counts significantly in some patients. Alan Jones suggests using the 30X potency three times daily over a period of four months.

ECHINACEA

Echinacea Angustifolia is well known for its bactericidal and fungicidal properties and is frequently used by people with HIV/AIDS as an adjunct to other therapeutic modalities. It purifies the blood, neutralises acids and removes toxins. *Echinacea* will be of service in many cases of septicaemia, especially where there is malignancy. Boils, carbuncles, abscesses, bad effects of vaccination. Mentally the patient is confused and depressed, cannot think clearly. Most often used in mother tincture or low potency.

GRAPHITES

Graphites was a remedy I rarely prescribed until I read Jan Scholten's[18] development of its central essence.

Patients who need this remedy are not always fat and slow although there is usually some kind of slowness about them, often as an intermediate state. For example, *Graphites* may be useful as an intercurrent remedy for a patient who is usually quick witted and clear thinking but who becomes dull, finding thinking difficult, which causes him to have doubts about himself.

Many HIV/AIDS patients naturally have these kinds of doubts, as if they lose contact with their central core essence which provides the meaning and values in their life. Scholten says that this can relate to an absent father or where the father's role has been unclear or weak. They do not know who the father really is or what he stands for and this makes them feel very anxious and unsure inside.

From my experience most gay men I have talked to have had a difficult or distant relationship with their father and so this remedy may be useful in some of these cases. (cf. *Calcarea Carbonica* and *Baryta Carbonica*.)

Graphites is also a big grief remedy. Interestingly, it is the only remedy listed under the rubric 'chronic grief' in *The Complete Repertory.* [19]

HYDRASTIS

Useful for pre- or post- cancerous conditions, as is well known, and also for infection states resulting in great loss of weight and weakness. It can help a patient to put on weight. Very good for cases of chronic constipation when other remedies don't work. Listed in *Murphy 's Repertory* [20] under obstinate constipation.

Cancer drainage: *Cundurango, Hydrastis, Gallium Apyrene*

KALI CARBONICA

I have treated only one case of acute PCP. This patient was a rigid, fearful person, quite reserved, and he had a dry tickling cough which made want to lean forwards with his elbows on his knees. *Kali Carbonica* certainly seemed to work before I lost touch with him.

LECITHIN

Lecithin is an important constituent in the vital processes of plant and animal organisms. Prepared from the yolk of an egg it is rich in phosphorus. *Lecithin* in potency has an affinity for the blood and positively influences the nutritive functions. Therefore it is useful in anaemia and in convalescence, especially where there is insomnia. In these cases it may be a good 'tonic' (cf. *Alfalfa*). The patient is tired, weak, short of breath with wasting. There is also mental exhaustion with forgetfulness, dullness and confusion.

LEPROMINIUM (Leprosy Nosode)

Although I have not had a chance to study the effects of *Leprominium*, I felt that a few details of this remedy, developed by Dr. Prakash Vakil, might be useful. Dr. Vakil speculates that :

> *"... leprosy affects the immune system very significantly over a period of time. This has led me to wonder whether the leprosy nosode might have a use in the treatment of immune disorders such as AIDS that are plaguing us in modern times."* [21]

People with leprosy and AIDS sufferers may share the following feelings about their disease and their relationship to society:

> *'Attributes the disease to fate. Feels no-one should suffer from such a disease. Feels dejected. In the initial stage, secludes himself, for he does not want others to know about his disease.'* (From the *Leprominium* proving).

The nosode has many skin symptoms which may indicate its use in some patients with Kaposi's sarcoma, especially with the characteristic general and mental symptoms.

LYCOPODIUM

This polychrest needs little mention save to say that it is extremely useful, together with *Carbo Vegetabilis*, where there is liver involvement. *Lycopodium* covers many AIDS type diseases well. It may be useful as a support remedy in the treatment of candidiasis (q.v.). I have also seen it do good work in the treatment of Kaposi's sarcoma lesions.

MEDORRHINUM

A very important remedy, especially in HIV+ cases before the onset of AIDS symptoms. In these cases *Medorrhinum* can help 'clear the ground' for further constitutional treatment. Such patients tend to be 'spaced out' with a history of recreational drugs, especially marijuana, and a wild lifestyle. I would go further and say that almost every patient I have treated who has taken many drugs (particularly marijuana) has benefited from *Medorrhinum* at some stage. There will often be frequent mood swings and an inability to 'get their life together'. Superficially, they may appear laid back but on closer questioning this may be due to a dope habit on which the patient depends to suppress anxiety. In comparison with *Tuberculinum, Medorrhinum* patients tend to be more weepy and sad, and less fiery.

A *Medorrhinum* medical history will often include multiple cases of gonorrhoea, syphilis and other types of venereal diseases, NSU, frequent colds with profuse catarrh, rheumatism, and all kinds of inflammations. Their family histories will frequently show early heart disease, arthritis, and mental problems like manic depression and alcoholism.

I often prescribe *Medorrhinum* in sequence with either *Thuja*, or *Carcinosin* and *Thuja* as an 'anti-sycotic'.

It is worth noting that a 'new version' of Medorrhinum, *Medorrhinum Americana* (named after the nationality of its donor), has recently become available.[22] It has received a combined meditative and conventional proving.[23] From the information received, it seems that *Medorrhinum Americana* may be especially suitable for people with HIV/AIDS as it presents a more syphilitic picture.

MERCURIUS CORROSIVUS

Similar to *Mercurius Solubilis* with salivation, sweating, weakness, but with more pain and destructiveness. Problems around the rectal area - abscesses, ulcers, bleeding, tenesmus. In other ways the picture looks like *Mercurius Solubilis* but in *Mercurius Corrosivus* the pain is the focus of the case. Affects all the mucous membranes.

One patient was rocking backwards and forwards on his chair as I took his case. He was HIV+ and was also haemophiliac, and was bleeding from the testicles into the scrotal sac. At first I thought of *Mercurius Solubilis* but on looking at the mental symptoms of *Mercurius Corrosivus*, I noticed 'Rocks hard'. It seemed like a remarkable symptom and indeed *Mercurius Corrosivus* worked wonders for this man. (For the rest of this case see section on Nosodes).

MERCURIUS SOLUBILIS

Patients needing *Mercurius Solubilis* can have a greasy, oily appearance, sometimes a slight yellowness. Mouth ulcers and receding or bleeding gums are common even to the extent of the teeth falling out. A good liver remedy, with pain and swelling. Stomach ulcers (I have found alternating *Mercurius* with *Kali Bichromicum* worked very well). Sinus problems. Post nasal catarrh. May be useful after abuse of antibiotics. All kinds of eye problems (ophthalmia, conjunctivitis, discharges, inflammations). Swelling of any or all glands. Vaginal herpes with discharge. Violence (may come out in dreams). I have often used it as a support remedy to treat an acute picture along with (for example) deeper miasmatic prescribing. Also remember the other *Mercury* salts (e.g. *Mercurius Iodatus Ruber* and *Mercurius Iodatus Flavus*).

Case: Male 37 yrs old. Short term memory loss for what he has just done. NBWS toxoplasmosis. Exhausted < slight exertion + palpitations. Short tempered. Fears snakes. Very jealous.

Rx: *Lachesis* and *Syphilinum* 1M (sequentially).

Good reaction but two months later came back with what appeared to be a return of toxoplasmosis: Very tired. Difficult visual co-ordination and judgement. Short term memory loss. Confused. Sweating and dribbling at night. Small ulcers on perianal tissue.

Rx: *Mercurius Sol* 10M.

Wonderful improvement! After that he needed *Calcarea Carbonica* and *Natrum Muriaticum* following which he looked almost like a different person!

MURIATIC ACID

'Hydrochloric acid has an elective affinity for the blood, producing septic conditions similar to that found in low fevers, with high temperature and great prostration',[24] says Phatak. Most of the acids have great prostration in their provings but none so great as *Muriatic Acid*, which 'slides down in bed'. We can therefore see the similarity with certain AIDS conditions, perhaps in the final stages. There is much muscular soreness, and (remembering that hydrochloric acid is a secretion of the stomach) the whole digestive tract is dry, bleeding, cracked and deeply ulcerated. *Muriatic Acid* is another remedy which may be useful in candidiasis where there is much weakness.

NATRUM SULPHURICUM

This remedy, as is well known, has a definite sycotic basis and, I believe, it may be an under used remedy. In any sycotic case think of *Natrum Sulphuricum* in the same way one might think of *Medorrhinum* or *Thuja*. Quite often it has proved of useful service when *Medorrhinum* or *Thuja* have seemed indicated but have failed. It may be useful in certain diarrhoea cases. The patient is often excessively gloomy and there may be a feeling of a loss of grace, beauty, or harmony. Many AIDS patients have this quality about them. Like many Thuja patients, those that need *Natrum Sulphuricum* often have a sense of 'unknowability'.

NITRICUM ACIDUM

Very anxious, together with a pronounced irritability.
Exceedingly chilly. Useful for rectal herpes, fistulas,
fissures and painful ulcers. I sometimes alternate with
Mercurius Corrosivus There is a feeling as if they are clinging
on to life and it is a battle. They hold onto everything -
'unforgiving'; even their stools! *Nitric Acidum* can look like
Arsenicum.

> **CASE:** Male 31 yrs. Presenting rectal ulcer since 6
> weeks with mucous discharge and terrible burning
> pain < night. Cannot sit (he lay on his side in the
> consulting room). Feet and hands very cold. Mollusci
> all over body. Tremendous anxiety and irritability with
> the pain.

> **Rx:** *Nitric Acid* and *Mercurius Corrosivus* 200
> Alternating doses, starting during consultation.

> By the end of the session the pain had receded to the
> extent that he could sit down! Over the next few
> months I continued treating him constitutionally but he
> always had his packets of *Nitric Acid* and *Mercurius
> Corrosivus* on him which he took as required. He
> returned once more the following year, having been
> basically well (the doctors were impressed!). This
> time he had become overheated whilst travelling in a
> hot climate and *Carbo Vegetabilis* was needed. I haven't
> seen him since.

Other *Nitricum* salts may prove useful (remember that Amyl
Nitrate is used by many as a recreational drug to enhance
dancing or sexual pleasure). If we consider how Nitrogen
itself is used in its frozen state to freeze off warts and
other skin lesions, is it too far fetched to consider using it
in homœopathic potency to do a similar job? Perhaps even
Kaposi's Sarcoma. could be treated in such a way. It has
been suggested[25] that *Nitrogen* (and *Carbon Dioxide)* could
help deal with the tubercular miasm.

PHOSPHORUS

Some of our best work can be done in helping patients to recover quickly following an acute episode.

CASE: Male 23 yrs. Had PCP 2 weeks previously. Taking high dose of Septrin which causes heartburn, migraines, nausea. He decides to stop the drug.
Now: Legs still weak < walking. Breathlessness walking long distances. Wants fish fingers, shellfish. Averse rich creamy sauces. Thirst for cold water. Has lost much weight - around two stones. Sweating at night profusely. Good energy. Blood-streaked mucus from nose. Nose blocked all the time.
Medical history: Recurrent tonsillitis, sore throats, bronchitis. Lot of penicillin, dope. Colds all year. Asthma. Gonorrhoea (few times)
Family: Lot of cancer

Rx: *Phosphorus* 12 tds for 7 days.

This young man appeared like a typical constitutional *Phosphorus* .

One week later he feels much better. There is a new symptom of a sensation of a hair on his tongue and the tongue is bright yellow.

Rx: *Natrum Phosphoricum* 6 tds for five days.

Thinking of all the antibiotics he had received plus his craving for fried fish (fish fingers) - *Natrum Phosphoricum* is good for excess acidity which often occurs after a course of antibiotics.

This cleared everything until **2 weeks later** when he was given Septrin prophylactically. He felt awful and developed candida, and was sweating profusely during the day.

Rx: *Natrum Phosphoricum* 1M plus
         China 6 tds (for fluid losses).

Five months later he reported a complete cessation
of all symptoms (including the oral hairy leukoplakia
which is a peculiar feature of AIDS).
A dose of *Phosphoric Acid* 200 was now needed,
however, following a bout of diarrhœa after drinking
some bad water.

Another case:
Male 49 yrs. History of Pneumonia, PCP, MAI. No energy.
Lost a good deal of weight. Not sleeping well.
Sensitive to light. Sensation as if oesophagus (perhaps
due to air tube damage) has narrowed, with difficulty
swallowing. Wounds slow to heal. Appetite poor. Very
thirsty. He says his positivity is waning. Walks with the
aid of a walking stick. Urination difficult, he never
feels finished.

Rx: *Phosphorus* 12 tds for seven days.

One week later: Much Better. Appetite very good. Can
walk without his stick. (Indeed he boasted how he had
run down the corridor earlier on!) Oesophagus
improved. Energy very good. Urinating without
difficulty.

Rx: *Tuberculinum* 200.

Frustratingly, the patient did not continue with treatment,
but I nevertheless felt pleased with the result.

PROTEUS

This bowel nosode deserves a separate note as I have found it so useful. It affects the nervous system, causing extreme tension and nervous exhaustion. The classic keyword associated with *Proteus* is 'brainstorm'. Patients who need *Proteus* are usually living in some kind of untenable situation: a woman who continues to work with her husband after he has gone off with another woman; businessmen working to impossible schedules; people who have been told they do not have long to live. Their nerves are stretched to their limits and the patient may appear as if they would explode with all the tension. So, one can see the relevance of *Proteus* to the HIV/AIDS condition, and many patients will benefit enormously from this remedy where the tension of living with the condition is uppermost. It especially corresponds with the emotional strains and social pressures of their situation.

It is also a useful remedy to give people who are on or have taken chemotherapy or other powerful drugs.

They have all kinds of cramps, numbness, paralysis, heartburn, indigestion and peptic ulcers. They may have cravings or aversions to butter, fats, pork, beef, eggs, onions, garlic, chocolate and sugar. Herpes, shingles or oedema can develop as a result of emotional strain. Recent cases of gonorrhoea treated with antibiotics may benefit from *Proteus.*

Proteus, when indicated, may have a wonderful calming effect on the patient. I most often use it to precede another related remedy.

Related remedies include: *Arsenicum, Anacardium, Nux Vomica, Thuja, Medorrhinum, Ignatia, Staphysagria.*

PYROGEN

Pyrogen can prove useful in ulcers, abscesses or bed sores where there are horribly foul smelling discharges.
I remember vividly one man I attended who had a necrotic cavity in his buttock. The smell was so putrid I felt quite nauseous. This patient needed *Pyrogen*. Any complaint where there is a suspected underlying septic focus may benefit from *Pyrogen*.

RADIUM BROMIDE

An often neglected remedy but, in my experience, an extremely useful one. I have used it successfully in cases of generalised weakness which have not responded to other indicated remedies. It may often be required in cases after drugging (esp. cortisones), where the body stores up toxicity in the joints causing stiffness and arthritic pains (> continued motion, like *Rhus Toxicodendron*). It can look like *Nux Vomica* in its irritability and like *Phosphorus* in its fears. It is also related to Pulsatilla in its craving for open air. Like X-ray it is often useful for the ill effects of radiation (cf. *Granite*). The ulceration it produces is similar to *Anacardium*.

RHUS TOXICODENDRON

An interesting remedy which can look like a cross between *Nitricum Acidum, Natrum Muriaticum,* and *Aurum* with much hopelessness and despair. *Rhus Tox*, however has more anguish and anxiety and restlessness. *Rhus Tox* fears death and thinks he is going to die, and has a strong anxiety for others e.g. her children.

There is also a little rubric which is quite useful - 'Delusion, that he is dirty' - in which *Rhus Tox* appears along with *Lac Caninum* and *Syphilinum*. I have treated patients who say their herpes make them feel dirty. *Rhus Tox* is a syphilitic remedy which is why it may be important in AIDS. A useful herpes remedy (Oral, genital or rectal - (cf. *Nitricum Acidum, Natrum Muriaticum*) also acute tonsillitis or influenza with extreme chilliness and restlessness (cf. *Arsenicum*).

Case: Severe depression. No reaction from 'common' depression remedies. < cloudy weather, autumn. *Rhus Tox* produced a positive reaction plus a recurrence of an old herpes lesion at the base of his spine.

If unsure of which remedy is indicated in acute herpes I may give may three remedies alternating in one day, e.g. *Natrum Muriaticum* or *Nitric Acid, Sulphur* and *Rhus Tox* .

STANNUM

Tremendous weakness. Sensation of hollowness in the chest. There may be sadness at not having achieved what they wanted to in life; they are discouraged; 'grief for the future'.

Stannum may look like *Natrum Muriaticum*. One patient I recall was undergoing psychotherapy and was examining his emotions a great deal. He felt tearful but found it difficult to express this - so it literally remained on his chest; he had also recently suffered PCP. He also had worms, another *Stannum* symptom. Although he had received other remedies, including *Natrum Muriaticum,* it was *Stannum* which helped him considerably.

SVA

There are various products on the market which claim to stimulate the immune function. One such product of possible interest to homœopaths is IMMUJEM-SVA-30[26] which is specifically for AIDS/AIDS-related conditions. According to Scott J. Gregory:

"SVA enhances the immune system and is anti-viral. It contains 8 homœopathic remedies. They are all in different dilutions, which were determined by much clinical experimentation. Every day's dosage and dilutions are different. The homœopathically potentised remedies in SVA include: RNA, Interleuken-I (locally short-acting hormone activating T4), Interleuken-III (hormone which stimulates all white blood cells), Interferon, hematopoetin (stimulates red blood cell production), PAA, and an immunoglobulin-g based broad spectral anti-viral." [27]

I mention this product because of its possible value in supplementing more individualised treatment.

SYPHILINUM

Black picture. Intense depression. Definite self-loathing. Fear is more self destructive; channelled into violence. Brain disorders. Can be very useful in cancer cases.

Some commentators, in particular Harris Coulter,[28] have drawn a link between syphilis and AIDS and, given the extremely destructive nature of both states this seems a fair assumption. Dr. Stephen Caiazza in New York noticed that almost all his AIDS patients tested positive for syphilis with the most sophisticated tests. He treated some 125 of these patients with penicillin, the conventional treatment for syphilis, with very positive results.[29]

The skin lesions associated with syphilis are very similar to

Kaposi's Sarcoma. Indeed, Moriz Kaposi first saw the skin condition which bears his name in a group of syphilitic patients. It is unlikely that syphilis is a major causative agent of AIDS; it is, however, one of a number of contributory factors.

THUJA

The sycotic miasm corresponds to the feeling of secrecy which many patients feel when they discover they are HIV+. They may not want their friends or relatives to know. They live a double life. Thus, *Thuja* is an important remedy here. Many gay people need *Thuja* because they feel distrust of a society which has seemingly rejected them. Inside they may feel guilty or shameful.They become doubtful of everything, even their own identity, and they may describe a feeling of detachment from the world. Several of my patients with AIDS have benefited from *Thuja* following vaccination. They often had not realised that the vaccinations were the cause of their decline in health; thus, it is always worth exploring vaccination histories carefully.

Thuja is a remedy which may prove useful constitutionally after acute herpes zoster (shingles). Patients who need *Thuja* may have oily skin and/or brittle hair.

THYMUS GLAND

Before approaching *Thymus Gland* as a remedy it is worth looking at the gland itself in a broader context. According to Barbara Brennan, in her book, *Light Emerging*,[30] the point in the upper chest where the thymus is situated, just beneath the upper part of the breastbone, is called the 'Soul Seat' in Eastern medicine. The Soul Seat relates to what a person wants to do in their life or the ability to look forward to a future; to form goals and to realise them. People who have problems with this centre may, according to Brennan, display a sunken chest and a give-up, 'I don't care', or a 'life is boring and meaningless' stance. They carry a deep sadness. One can therefore see how this might correlate with people with HIV/AIDS. The moment such people have been given an HIV label, life suddenly collapses or is reduced to a day-by-day existence with no broader vision. So, the thymus gland relates in some way to a person's vision of life.

One of the strange properties of the thymus gland, in response to acute stress, is that it may shrivel to half its size in just twenty-four hours. A large thymus gland in children was at one time thought to be implicated in 'crib death'.

The effectiveness, or otherwise, of the thymus gland may have a relationship to cancerous growth. In the embryo and early life the thymus affects physical growth and later matures the lymphocytes which give rise to the T-cells. These then leave the thymus and travel to the lymph nodes and spleen where they become responsible for the processes of immunity in the body. The departed T-cells, however, are still influenced by the thymus which continues to send hormones through the bloodstream. After puberty the thymus *should* shrink in size as its job concerning growth has now finished but if it fails to atrophy this may indicate a block in the sexual maturing process.

John Diamond,[31] who has researched into the emotions connected with the different organs of the body, says that the thymus is connected with love, faith, gratitude, trust and courage in its positive mode, and hate, fear and envy in the negative. One HIV+ patient I recall, indeed, had an interesting reaction to *Thymus Gland* in potency. He reported, after taking it, that for the first time he could imagine being totally well. Another patient told me that she was sleepless due to an upsurge in her energy levels. I have given the remedy to other people with some good results but there obviously needs to be further exploration.

Colin Griffiths together with a group of homœopaths in South London have carried out some highly interesting research through clinical observations and an informal meditative proving[32] into *Thymus Gland* as a remedy. Griffiths gives the following information:

> *"Damage to the thymus gland can be caused by severe trauma, mechanical accident and immunisation; drug intervention (particularly antibiotics and steroids) and emotional trauma in children especially if sustained for any length of time, is certain to affect this gland; fearfulness that induces emotional dependency is a prime indication. In adults this often becomes fear of disease with a dependency on medical intervention....."*

> *".......frequent acute illnesses which affect the lungs, mucous membranes, liver (fevers) and bowels; inexplicable weight gains, losses or swings; they are cut off from any family tradition, no sense of continuity; they seem unaware of their raison d'être....as if they function unquestioningly; despair of recovery, hopeless, despondent; deep hurt which they cannot express; sense of disorientation, of being spaced out or far off; sense of insecurity; afraid of being hurt; afraid of meeting new challenges in case success should cause them to feel independent; one who has been emotionally/spiritually damaged and who is left without a place or purpose."*

Thymus Gland can be prescribed in various ways: as a remedy in its own right; as a drainage remedy to support the action of the chosen main remedies (for example, in 6X or 6C once or twice daily); as part of a combination, again, as a support.

With respect to the latter, Griffiths gives three examples which, in my opinion, may be useful in AIDS cases:

1. Thymus gland + Arsenicum Album + Syphilinum
Long standing sense of guilt. Identity crisis; feel desperately confused and lost - their purpose is temporarily removed from sight; they need reassurance and easily become dependent on therapist. Underlying all this is a sense of facing the abyss. This combination has been observed to be profoundly relaxing. Can be useful, according to Martin Miles, for suspected PCP- this combination 'takes it off the chest'.

2. Thymus gland + Ignatia + Tuberculinum
For those who apparently need *Natrum Muriaticum* but who have not responded particularly well. The patient recognises degree of effort needed to effect an emotional change and shies away from it. This combination can help them to recognise what hurt needs to be addressed, accepted and healed.

3. Thymus gland + Ignatia + Syphilinum
Acute grief in those who keep suffering emotional blows. Helps to break the pattern. Can be used in chronic cases where the main remedy has uncovered a well of grief which the patient would prefer not to handle.

TUBERCULINUM

The tubercular miasm may be seen in many aspects of HIV/AIDS. Many of the physical conditions associated with AIDS are related to the lungs. A number of patients even develop TB itself (in AIDS patients tuberculosis is six times more common than in the general population).

People who need *Tuberculinum* often have a sense of being driven. There is a strong desire to experience life to extremes with the result that they burn out. It is then that the respiratory diseases appear. It is a great remedy for night sweats and will often relieve debility in appropriate cases.

Useful in a history of TB , PCP, tonsillitis, bronchitis and recurring upper respiratory tract infections. Strengthens the whole chest area. No appetite with wasting. Night sweats and fevers (cf. *Mercurius*). Generalised lymphatic involvement with swollen glands.

Consider *Tuberculinum Aviare* where there is acute influenza bronchitis with symptoms similar to TB, e.g. debility, diminished appetite and an incessant, irritating or tickling cough.

TYPHOIDINUM

Alan Jones says:

"There is very little data on provings of Typhoidinum, but comparison of the clinical symptoms of typhoid & AIDS show a marked similarity. They are both characterised by reduction in WBC count, oral 'thrush', abdominal bloating with diarrhœa, splenomegaly, and dark red-purple ulcerating skin lesions. Used in the 30X-200X potency range, Typhoidinum has given reasonable increases in T4 cell count and T4/T8 ratios, and can be used as an alternative to the Cyclosporin/Thymosin regime."

Rajan Sankaran in *The Substance of Homœopathy* has a picure of Typhoidinum.[33]

VANADIUM METALLICUM

This was another remedy to come to my attention through Jan Scholten's book.[34] Certainly when I had looked through its fairly brief symptom picture I was struck by its similarity to the AIDS condition: degenerative conditions with softening of the brain, anaemia, emaciation, TB, neuro-retinitis and blindness (CMV). Scholten cites his use of it in cases of anorexia or bulimia. There is also a repeated failure pattern in such patients. They have a great need to succeed in their undertakings but they have low expectations of themselves and this need is often related to the expectations of a dominant parent figure.

Case: Female 25 yrs: HIV+
She has been in therapy for over 2 yrs. She has experienced sleeplessness for 4 months since visiting parents.
She says she has many issues around abuse - anger, tears, breathlessness, sighing, sadness. Feels vulnerable. Dreams of being naked while trying to express herself. Wakes feeling angry, irritable. Was raped in 1989 (for the first time), but has always been scared of boys. Very analytical. She has a 'given up' look, sunken chest, small child-like voice (*Thymus gland?*) and appears as if she feels a failure. Used to be addicted to drugs and alcohol; also suffers from bulimia/anorexia. Fear of failure. Fear of what people will think of her- that she is not strong or cannot handle things. She feels deep shame. Father was a military man-very dominant. She is tired, listless, aching muscles. Eczema on face, cysts on neck.

Rx: *Vanadium* 9c bd for one week then *Vanadium* 1M

One of the aspects in HIV/AIDS cases is often a deep sense of failure, they have failed society. So they give up, it's as if they are going to die anyway, so what's the point. This can look like the *Vanadium* picture.

2 weeks later:
She was much improved. Much higher energy, more
passionate about life, sleep >, skin >. So many plans
and ideas she does not know how to channel energy.

Rx: *Calcarea Phosphorica* 1M

Based on restlessness, desire to travel, fear of being
judged (i.e. insecurity) on her opinions and a definite
tubercular appearance. She did very well on this and other
remedies, really getting her life together.

This idea of a dominant parent figure in *Vanadium* seems
very important and is so common in my experience, as is
the sense of a lack of identity. Interestingly this is
reflected in the nature of the element itself. Vanadium
exists in five different oxidation states and will freely
change from one to another. The salts formed in each state
are all of different colours. In industry it is used as a
catalyst, and as an oxidising agent - it being freely reduced
by more dominant agents, and it is added to steel to make
it more flexible.

Other keynote symptoms of Vanadium include:

Dream/delusion/sensation of missing the boat/train.
Craving for liquorice
Aggravation at the time of ovulation
Ailments dating from puberty

I have treated other anorexic, bulimic, addictive patients
with this remedy with good results. Whether or not it
would be useful in gross AIDS pathology remains to be
seen. *Vanadium* is another remedy which seems to have an
affinity with the thymus gland and I have used *Thymus Gland*
in a low potency (e.g. 6c once a day) to support the action
of the *Vanadium* with very positive results.

Vanadium resembles several other hysteria remedies:
Pulsatilla, Ignatia, Staphysagria, Anacardium, Carcinosin.

X-RAY

Potentially this may be a very useful remedy for all kinds of immune disorders. Boericke[35] says of *X-ray* ".....*it brings to the surface suppressed symptoms.....*"

Allen has the following to say:

> "*When the sycotic or syphilitic virus is grafted on a psoric or tubercular diathesis; when from the paucity of presenting symptoms it is almost impossible to be certain of the predominant diathesis, in consequence of which the best selected antipsoric, Calcarea, Medorrhinum, Psorinum, Sepia, Sulphur, Syphilinum, or Tuberculinum, fails to relieve or to rouse the overpowered vitality to a sufficient degree to throw off or bring to the surface the predominant toxin, the X-ray bids fair to be our curative remedy.*"[36]

X rays can definitely impair immune function. They may have a very specific effect on the thymus gland, in which case *X-ray* and *Thymus Gland* in potency may work well together.

It may be of use where there is an old unresolved inflammation that continues in a low-level way e.g. burns and ulcers that refuse to heal. Murphy[37] mentions low vitality, chronic fatigue, unexplained weakness, general debility and "patients submitted for therapy by immuno-suppressors and all anti-tumour chemotherapy." X-ray can be thought of as an 'auto-immune nosode', especially where the person is overly concerned with environmental triggers such as pollution, geopathic stress, food additives etc. These people may be of a hypochondriacal nature and their life may have contracted to the point where their poor health has become the dominating feature - everything affects them negatively; they have no broader vision of their life cf.*Thymus Gland.*

A Medical Overview Of Aids

(Julie Williams)

Since the advent of AIDS, epidemiologists have speculated on its origins. The theories proliferate each year, ranging from a connection to the smallpox vaccine to cross-species infection from monkeys to man following trials of a polio vaccine in the 1920's.

AIDS is an immune deficiency state in which a particular sub-group of lymphocytes, known as T4 or CD4 cells, are particularly affected. Viruses are inactive chemical substances which have no reproductive or metabolic capacity. They consist of a core containing genetic material and an enzyme (reverse transcriptase). This is coated with proteins and a fatty membrane. In order to multiply, the virus has to invade host cells and utilise *their* reproductive abilities.

Human Immunodeficiency Virus (HIV) is from a sub family of 'retroviruses'. These convert their own RNA into a 'recombinant' DNA which integrates with the host cell's DNA to produce an entirely different 'viral-cell', and this results in an infection of indefinite duration. This alien cell remains dormant until attacked by an antigen, usually a cytomegalovirus or herpes virus, which causes the DNA to replicate rapidly. This is similar to an allergic reaction and it ends up killing the cell. HIV will only infect cells which have the right 'receptors' on their surface, the Helper T lymphocytes (CD4 or T4 cells) and cells of the central nervous system.

T4 cells are central to the normal functioning of the immune system. They 'recognise' foreign antigens and stimulate production of B cells which produce antibodies which, in turn, kill the invaders. T4 cells also stimulate cell-mediated immunity in which infected cells are destroyed by cytotoxic cells (T8 and NK cells). Hence, the T4, T8 cell counts and the ratio of T4:T8 cells are used as an indication of the extent of opportunistic infection. Antibody-mediated immunity, on the other hand, relies on antibody, rather than T cell, production. Thus bacterial infections are not generally problematical in T-cell reduced situations. Of crucial interest to homœopaths is the fact that the HIV will only develop in the right environment. In this sense it is opportunistic.

The result of infection by HIV is a highly increased susceptibility to infections, especially viral and fungal ones, and also an increased susceptibility to certain types of cancer. Someone whose immune system is compromised in this way can be severely affected by an infection which would be mild or go unnoticed in a healthy person. Such infections are described as 'opportunistic'.

The conventional belief is that AIDS is related, in whole or in part, to infection with HIV. This view has been questioned, and the resulting debate is highly contentious - but that is too large a subject to address here. It suffices to say that various co-factors are thought to play some part in the speed and progress of the disease.

HIV infection is spread through the exchange of body fluids with an infected person. This means that it can be transmitted sexually; through injecting equipment and contaminated blood; and from mother to child during pregnancy. Presumably babies remain at risk due to the immaturity of their immune systems.

The HIV test detects the presence of antibodies to HIV in the blood. A positive result means that there has been contact with HIV. It is not known what proportion of those who are HIV positive (HIV+) will go on to develop AIDS. To test HIV+ is not the same as a diagnosis of AIDS. Moreover,

in the first few weeks or months after exposure, antibodies
will not yet have been produced, and the test will be
negative. During this time there may or may not be
symptoms of 'acute seroconversion illness' with fever,
fatigue and flu-like symptoms.

This initial stage usually resolves and there follows a
period of variable length, but sometimes ten years or more,
without symptoms. Various symptoms can be associated
with 'HIV disease' which are not sufficient in themselves to
constitute a diagnosis of AIDS:

• **Profound and persistent fatigue with no obvious
  cause**
• **Unexplained weight loss (more than ten pounds in
  two months)**
• **Recurrent drenching night sweats**
• **Fevers of unknown origin, lasting in excess of ten
  days**
• **Persistent diarrhœa**
• **Enlarged lymph glands (PGL - persistent generalised
    lymphadenopathy)**
• **Seborrheic dermatitis**
• **Post-nasal drip**
• **Increased severity of warts or herpes**
• **Menstrual irregularities and persistent vaginal
  infections**

The diagnosis of AIDS was originally made if one or more of
a list of recognised opportunistic infections occurred.
As experience of treating this condition increased, the list
grew longer and longer. Then the Centre for Disease
Control (CDC) in America introduced a new diagnostic
criterion: a CD4 count below 200 was considered indicative
of AIDS. This measure is controversial: on the one hand it is
an objective measure which is easy to apply but there is no
absolute correlation between the CD4 count and a person's
state of health.

Someone whose immune system is compromised and who has increased susceptibility to infection can potentially be susceptible to an extremely wide range of disorders, so the clinical manifestations of AIDS are myriad. They can include infection with a number of unusual organisms seldom seen otherwise, and accurate diagnosis can be difficult or elusive. As well as infections, there can also be malignancies and blood disorders. While there is no typical pattern of this disease, there are some diseases and symptoms frequently associated with AIDS which will be seen regularly by someone practising in this field of medicine.

Respiratory disorders are the most common manifestations of AIDS. Over 60% of patients have at least one such episode during the course of their disease, most commonly coughs and shortness of breath, with or without fever and sweats. The most common causes include: Pneumocystis Carinii Pneumonia (PCP), Cytomegalovirus, Kaposi's Sarcoma (q.v.), Pneumococcus.

One of the most frequent 'AIDS indicator diseases' is **Pneumocystis Carinii Pneumonia** (PCP) which produces severe shortness of breath and dry unproductive coughs. This can be a serious infection for which the favoured medical treatment is high-dose Septrin (co-trimoxazole). Prophylactic drug treatment is recommended if there has already been an episode of PCP, or if the CD4 count is low. This may involve a lower dose of Septrin, or inhaled Pentamidine as an alternative. Septrin is regarded as the most effective treatment, but also the most toxic. The main side effects are nausea and vomiting, rash, and bone marrow toxicity resulting in leucopenia. This last is particularly problematic if Zidovudine (AZT) is also being taken. Pentamidine if inhaled can cause cough, bronchoconstriction and metallic taste in the mouth. If given intravenously it can cause renal toxicity or a fall in blood pressure and/or blood glucose levels.

Tuberculosis is six times more common amongst those who are HIV+, compared with the general population. Treatment is the same as in any case of TB. It is thought that TB may accelerate the progress of HIV disease.

Chest infection with another Mycobacterium, **Mycobacterium avium intracellulare** (MAI) can also occur, especially later in the course of the disease. Generalised as well as respiratory symptoms are seen here: fever, sweats, weight loss, loss of appetite, anaemia, lymphadenopathy.

The gastro-intestinal tract is another site for many AIDS-related symptoms: in the oropharynx, **Candidiasis** (thrush), **hairy leukoplakia, ulcers, abscesses** and **gum disease** may occur; thrush may spread from the mouth into the throat and then into the oesophagus, causing difficulty in swallowing and retrosternal pain, as well as the characteristic white spots in the mouth. If this is a recurrent problem, or immunocompromise is severe, anti-fungal drugs such as Ketoconazole may be prescribed prophylactically. Some of these require tests to monitor liver function.

Chronic **diarrhoea** is a common problem in HIV disease, whether AIDS defined or not. Wasting may well be seen alongside the diarrhoea, caused by fluid loss and malabsorption of food . It can be difficult to identify a causative organism, which means that treatment will focus on symptomatic relief rather than specific anti-microbial activity. One of the opportunistic causes of such disease is the protozoan, cryptosporidium.

Skin conditions are common and may be severe at all stages of HIV disease, as previously mentioned. These may include herpes simplex, warts (human papilloma virus), varicella zoster (shingles), molluscum contagiosum, tinea (ringworm), candidiasis, folliculitis, seborrheic dermatitis and psoriasis. They may appear for the first time or be an exacerbation of a pre-existing condition.

Kaposi's sarcoma is a malignant vascular tumour which resembles a raised bruise. The lesions are firm painless nodules of a dark red or purple colouration. Before the advent of AIDS, it was usually seen in elderly Jewish men and in the inhabitants of sub-Saharan Africa. Although usually identified by its skin lesions, it can also affect internal organs, particularly the gastro-intestinal tract and lungs. The appearance of the lesions may be unsightly and give rise to anxiety about appearance.

Enlarged lymph glands may occur as a generalised response to the condition itself; be related to specific infections, e.g. TB; or be a result of malignant lymphomas. Aggressive tumours of the lymphatic systems - usually non Hodgkin's lymphoma - are one of the most common malignancies associated with AIDS. The lymph nodes themselves may enlarge enormously, multiple sites may be involved, and these may metastasize to the brain, producing neurological symptoms.

Retinitis, with or without **encephalitis**, may occur, associated with the cytomegalovirus (CMV). This produces severe and progressive visual impairment. The infection is chronic, and allopathic treatment, once initiated, continues for life. Headache and confusion suggest the onset either of encephalitis or of a brain abscess. There may also be convulsions, personality changes and specific neurological signs such as hemiplegia. Encephalitis may be due to CMV or to toxoplasmosis. Similar symptoms are produced by cerebral lymphoma.

Meningitis can be caused by the fungus Cryptococcus neoformans. This may sometimes lack the classic symptom of neck stiffness, the main symptoms being malaise, headache and fever. Treatment is with antifungal drugs such as amphotericin.

The primary disease condition can itself lead to dementia, usually at a late stage of progression. Patients become confused, disorientated, apathetic, emotionally unresponsive and lacking in concentration and memory. This state can resemble the effects of infections such as pneumonia, or of the drugs used to treat them, and emotional states such as depression.

Medical Tests And Drugs

T4 (CD4) Lymphocyte Count

Many HIV/AIDS patients are tested regularly to determine their T4 lymphocyte count, which the medical profession employs as one measure of the strength of a person's immune system. It is also used by doctors to determine whether a person should be prescribed AZT (where the T4 cell count is lower than 500). Basically, the higher the count the healthier the person is supposed to be. A normal count is above 1000, some people with HIV have a count of ten or less. A modern diagnosis of AIDS is made when a person has a T4 cell count less than 200.

In reality there are people who are relatively healthy with a T4 count of three and people with 300 who are quite sick. So the T4 cell count is not in itself an accurate measure of health. One problem is that the lymphocyte levels may be sensitive to the mood changes of the patient, e.g. anxiety and stress. Often when patients go for a test their acute anxiety has negative effects on the result. Of course, these results may then further damage the patient's morale if they seem to indicate a downward trend.

If a patient seems badly affected by these procedures, it could be justifiably asked who benefits from them. Many patients have made the choice to discontinue the monthly T4 cell counts with no seeming disadvantage.

DRUGS

Drugs used in AIDS-related conditions can be used either:
specifically against the HIV virus; to treat opportunistic
infections that have occurred; as prophylaxis of common
opportunistic infections; or as treatment for pre-existing
conditions.

Of the anti-HIV drugs, Zidovudine (AZT) is the most widely
used at present. AZT inhibits the HIV virus but does not
eradicate it from the body; hence it is not expected to cure
AIDS, only to slow the progress of the disease. The main
side-effects of AZT are haematological. This toxicity may
be so severe as to prevent some people from taking this
drug, or to require blood transfusions. Liver function can
also be affected adversely. Other side effects can include:
loss of appetite, digestive disturbances, malaise, fatigue,
insomnia, fever, myopathy, neuropathy.

Recently, cocktails of drugs including AZT, DDI, Acyclovir
and others have been the preferred course of treatment as,
in allopathic terms, they have been observed to be more
effective.

In the case of opportunistic infections, by definition, a
broad variety of these may occur in those living with AIDS
so the range of drugs used to treat them will be similarly
broad. Disease patterns seems to vary in different affected
groups, e.g. gay men, women, Africans.

When treating patients from Africa be sure to ask about
any history of malaria in their early life. Such patients have
often received frequent courses of Chloroquin which is
prescribed as abundantly in Africa as antibiotics are in the
West, and which can be very toxic and damaging. The
combination of chronic malaria and extensive drugging may
form another pathology layer which will need to be
addressed during homœopathic treatment.

Septrin, which is a commonly used prophylactic against PCP, is a powerful antibiotic with numerous severe side effects. In my experience, Septrin tends to interfere with the effect of homœopathic remedies. Two patients who had responded well to remedies saw their symptoms return when they started taking Septrin. Moreover, in active PCP the dosage of Septrin prescribed is considerably higher (normally over three times) than that which is usual in other acute conditions.

Many patients will be taking a large number of drugs when they present, and in many different combinations. This can obviously present a challenge to homœopathic treatment. The drugs prescribed to people with HIV/AIDS can have a number of negative effects, from a homœopathic point of view:

- **They can mask or suppress the true symptom picture**
  In these cases it may be necessary to trace back to the original symptom picture prior to taking the drugs. However, if a drug or drugs are powerful enough to suppress the true symptom picture they will frequently interfere with the action of the homœopathic remedies. In which case homœopathic treatment may prove difficult without bringing the patient off the offending drugs. Such drugs include morphine and derivatives, cortisones, Septrin and other broad-spectrum antibiotics.

- **They can cause their own side effects**
  If a drug is causing side effects (and this may be difficult to discern, given the number of drugs patients with AIDS are often taking, and the frequent complexity of the symptom picture), prescribing the drug in potency (for example, a 30c repeated over 2-3 days) may be useful. In addition, or as a substitute, one could try *Nux Vomica* alternating with *Sulphur* or *Pulsatilla* in a low potency repeated over a few days. This has a detoxifying or blood-cleansing effect. *Okoubaka*[38] is a relatively recent

addition to our materia medica which may be useful
where there are effects from drugging with allergic
reactions. *Opium* is good for constipation in heroin
addicts and can be prescribed as they withdraw from the
drug. It also clears the mind. Alternatively, a combination
of *Nux Vomica, Bryonia* and *Opium* may work wonders
and has the added benefit of stimulating the liver. *China*
is a useful remedy for diarrhoea following antibiotics.

• **They can deplete the energy level**
This may be due to the effect they have on the endocrine
system, for example the thyroid, and other organs.
Sometimes an endocrine stimulant (e.g. *Thyroidinum/Fucus
Vesiculosus/Iodum*) in low potency, repeated, can be
useful. A nosode such as *Medorrhinum* may be needed.
X- ray after radio- or chemo-therapy and *Thymus Gland*
after vaccination in homœopathic potency have
sometimes proved their worth in this regard. Consider
general tonics such as *Avena Sativa* and *Alfalfa* in a
mother tincture, especially after morphine based drugs.

• **They can cause congestion in various organs**
Congestion or damage of the body's organs leads to an
inability to eliminate toxins, to adequately process foods
within the system, or to deal with stress. Steroids, in
particular, may be very damaging in this regard; long term
usage atrophies the adrenal cortex. People who are
stopping their steroid drugs will often benefit from a
course of *Adrenal Cortex* or *A.C.T. Hormone* in a low (e.g.
6c) potency. There are various liver support remedies: a
combination of *Chelidonium, Hydrastis* and *Carduus
Marianus* (or *Nux Vomica*) is very useful. A few doses of
Liver 30c is another possibility.

• **They can interfere with the internal environment**
Leading to local or systemic candidiasis (or other yeast-
based/protozoal infections)
There are various naturopathic and homœopathic
solutions to these problems. Isopathic preparation of the

yeast or protozoan concerned may be useful. See the section on Candida for more information.

Where one particular drug, e.g. Penicillin, has been taken over a long period of time , it is certainly worth, and in many cases important and necessary, to give the drug in a high potency in order to detoxify the body. Frequently the patient is proving that drug.

There are often thorny emotional issues for patients who are taking drugs. Many patients face pressure from family, friends and doctors to take the allopathic drugs so that a real choice in the matter becomes difficult. Much of the problem centres around how secure or safe the patient feels. Sometimes patients feels that if they commit themselves to the homœopathic approach this will be a one-way street, so as to speak, which is obviously not the case. The solution I believe is to educate the patient and provide a safe environment so that he or she can make a considered choice. In the final analysis, the most important consideration is the patient's ability to feel in control of his or her life.

Of course it may prove impossible to treat patients homœopathically who are taking large amounts of medical drugs. Generally speaking, the more apparent or clear the original symptom picture -in spite of drugging - the easier is the treatment. Frequently, there may only be an unclear picture to treat and this will often present greater difficulties.

If you do feel moved to treat a patient who is taking powerful drugs such as morphine or steroids you might consider creating a 'window' for the indicated remedy by prescribing the drug in potency just before the indicated remedy. It is often best in these cases to repeat the indicated remedy at frequent intervals, preceding each dose with the potentised drug. LM potencies are especially suitable. Remember that drugs often present another layer which may have to be dealt with separately.

MEDICAL DRUGS COMMONLY
USED IN TREATMENT OF HIV/AIDS[39]

1=Use
2=Side effects
3= Homœopathic compatability

ACYCLOVIR
1. Antiviral. Treats infection by herpes virus (e.g.. shingles, genital herpes). Can be used prophylactically. Orally, topically or intravenously.
2. Orally; gastrointestinal disturbance, blood cell deficiencies, fatigue, rash, headaches, tremor, mood changes.
3. OK where no side effects apparent.

AZT (aka Zidovudine)
1. Antiviral. Main anti-HIV drug. Orally or intravenously.
2.Affects production of red and white blood cell production, bone marrow, blood transfusions often required, nausea and vomiting, gastrointestinal disturbances, loss of appetite, headache, rashes, fever, sleep disturbances.
3. OK where no side effects apparent.

CLINDAMYCIN
1.Antibacterial. Treats toxoplasmosis and other infections. Orally or intravenously.
2. Diarrhoea, colitis, nausea, vomiting, abdominal discomfort, jaundice, liver dysfunction, blood disorders.
3. Difficult.

CODEINE PHOSPHATE (similar to DF 118)
1. Opioid narcotic analgesic. Also anti-diarrhoeal. Treats
mild to moderate pain and diarrhoea. Orally or by injection.
2. Nausea and vomiting, loss of appetite, urinary retention,
constipation, mood changes, confusion, dry mouth,
flushing of face, sweating, headache, palpitations, postural
hypotension (dizziness on standing), slowed heart rate.
3. Difficult.

DAPSONE
1.Antibacterial. Commonly used to treat malaria, leprosy
and tuberculosis.
AIDS: treats PCP usually when patient is allergic to Septrin.
Orally or intravenously.
2. Nausea, vomiting, headache, insomnia, increased heart
rate, severe weight loss, anaemia, hepatitis, peripheral
nerve damage, blood changes.
3. OK where no side effects apparent.

DDC (aka Zalcitabine)
1. Antiviral. For patients who are intolerant to, or have not
responded to AZT. Orally.
2. Peripheral neuropathy, nausea, vomiting, mouth ulcers,
anorexia, diarrhoea, constipation, abdominal pain,
headache, dizziness, rashes.
3. OK where side effects not apparent.

DDI (aka Didanosine)
1. Antiviral. For patients who are intolerant to, or have not
responded to AZT. Orally.
2. Pancreatitis, peripheral neuropathy, raised blood urea
levels, nausea, vomiting, confusion, fever and headache.
3. OK where side effects not apparent.

FLUCONAZOLE
1. Antifungal. Treats many fungal infections including candidiasis of mucous membranes-vagina, mouth, oesophagus, athlete's foot, cryptococcal meningitis. Orally or intravenously.
2. Nausea, abdominal discomfort, flatulence, diarrhoea, headaches, rash, angio-oedema, anaphylaxis, alteration of liver enzymes.
3. OK where no side effects apparent.

GANCICLOVIR
1. Antiviral. Treats cytomegalovirus infection of eyes and intestines. Intravenously.
2. Blood disorders, sore throat, swelling of face, fever, rash, disturbs liver function, G.I. tract disturbances.
3. OK where no side effects apparent.

KETOCONAZOLE
1. Treats deep-seated and serious fungal infections esp. candidiasis. Orally or topically.
2. Serious liver damage, itching rash, abdominal pain, blood disorders, breast enlargement in men.
3. OK where no side effects apparent.

PENTAMIDINE
1. Antiprotozoal. Treats PCP, either intravenously or inhalation.
2. Severe hypotension, pancreatitis, hypoglycaemia, arrhythmia, blood disorders, kidney failure.
3. OK where no side effects apparent.

PYREMETHAMINE
1. Antiprotozoal, antimalarial. Treats toxoplasmosis together with Sulphadiazine. Orally.
2. Rashes, insomnia, blood disorders.
3. Difficult.

SEPTRIN (aka Co-trimoxazole)
1. Antibacterial/antiprotozoal. Main drug for treatment of PCP. Intravenous or orally.
2. Nausea and vomiting, diarrhoea, rashes, blood disorders. In a few cases has caused fatal allergic reaction.
3. Difficult.

SULPHADIAZINE
1. Antibacterial. Treats toxoplasmosis together with Pyremethamine. Orally or intravenously.
2. Nausea and vomiting, diarrhoea, rashes, blood disorders. In a few cases has caused fatal allergic reaction.
3. Difficult.

Other drugs with limited homœopathic compatibility include: corticosteroids, morphine based drugs (including DF118 painkillers), TB drugs (e.g. Rifanal and others), antidepressants and antiepileptics (e.g. Phenytoin).

In Conclusion

*"The highest ideal of cure is rapid, permanent,
restoration of the health or removal and annihilation of
the disease in its whole extent, in the most reliable and
most harmless way on easily comprehensible principles"* [40]

Samuel Hahnemann

**So what hope *is* there for people suffering with AIDS
using alternative approaches?**

First, it should be noted that from a survey carried out at a
major HIV/AIDS centre in London, most people indicated
that it was the *alternative* therapies, freely provided, which
drew them to use the Centre regularly.

Secondly, AIDS has clearly attracted a panoply of
alternative therapists and treatments, all offering their
individual approaches, which, in itself, may further confuse
those seeking solutions.

Over the four years I spent treating people with HIV/AIDS I
saw many people helped by a range of approaches, some
dramatically. At one point I carried out an approximate
audit of my own cases and found that around 50% had been
at least helped by homœopathy and some of these made
significant improvements in their condition.

As I have already indicated, I believe homœopathy has a
major part to play in the treatment of AIDS. Indeed, the
failure of mainstream Western medicine to convincingly
offer a solution which does not further harm the immune
system and which honours the integrity of the individual
would seem to make homœopathy deserving of serious
consideration and further research.

Adler, Michael W. (ed.)
ABC of AIDS, 3rd edition, BMJ, London 1993.
Barker, Raymond Charles
Treat Yourself to Life, Perigree Books,
New York 1991
Brennan, Barbara Ann
Hands of Light, Bantam, New York 1988.
Light Emerging, Bantam, New York 1993.
Burnett, James Compton.
Best of Burnett, (ed. Chitkara), B. Jain Publishers
Pvt. Ltd, New Delhi 1992.
Chaitow, Leon and Simon Martin
A World Without AIDS, Thorsons, Wellingborough
1988.
Coulter, Harris
Syphilis and AIDS, B Jain Publishers Pvt. Ltd, New
Delhi, India
Diamond, John
Life Energy, Paragon House, New York 1985.
Your Body Doesn't Lie, Warner Books, New York
1979.
Eisayaga, F
Treatize on Homœopathic Medicine, Ediciones
Marecel, Buenos Aires 1994
Grossinger, Richard
Planet Medicine, 5th edition, North Atlantic Books,
Berkeley 1990.
Gregory, Scott J.
A Holistic Protocol for the Immune System **(6th)**
Tree of Life Publications (PO Box 126, Joshua Tree,
CA 92252, USA), 1995
Hahnemann, Samuel
Organon of Medicine, 6th Edit., Victor Gollancz,
London 1983.
Handley, Rima
A Homœopathic Love Story, North Atlantic,
Berkeley , Calif. 1990
MacDonald-Bayne, Murdo
Spiritual and Mental Healing, Fowler, Romford,
Essex 1947

McTaggart, Lynne (ed.)
What Doctors Don't Tell You, 4 Wallace Road,
London.
Morton, Dr Ian and Dr Judith Hall,
Medicines-The Comprehensive Guide, 3rd Edition,
Bloomsbury, London 1995
Murphy R
Lotus Materia Medica, Lotus Star Academy,
Colorado USA 1995
Phatak, Dr. S R
Materia Medica, Indian Books and Periodicals
Syndicate, New Delhi, India
Sakoian, Francis and Louis S. Acker
T he Astrologer's Handbook, Penguin , 1981.
Sankaran, Rajan
The Spirit of Homoeopathy, Dr Rajan Sankaran,
Bombay 1991.
The Substance of Homoeopathy,
Homœopathic Medical Publishers, Bombay 1994.
Scholten, Jan.
Homoeopathy and Minerals, Stichting Alonnissos,
Utrecht 1993.
Serinus, Jason (ed.)
Psychoimmunity & The Healing Process,
3rd ed., Celestial Arts, Berkeley 1988.
Steinbrecher, Edwin C.
The Inner Guide Meditation, The Aquarian Press,
Wellingborough 1982.
Vermeulen, Frans.
Concordant Materia Medica, Merlijn Publishers,
Haarlem 1994.
Weeks, Nora
Medical Discoveries of Edward Bach, C.W. Daniel
Co. Ltd., Saffron Walden, Essex
Williams, Ian and Adrian Mindel and Ian V.D. Weller.
AIDS, Gower Medical Publishing, London 1989
Zandvoort, Roger van
Complete Repertory of the Mind, I R H I S,
Leidschendam, Holland

Useful Addresses

The following list is a selection of resource agencies which can offer advice, information and, in some cases, counselling and holistic treatments. They should, at the very least, be able to refer enquirers on to other appropriate organisations. It is not complete, and while all details have been verified with the National AIDS Manual, there may be errors due to the shifting nature of client needs, funding and other imponderables.

There are relatively few homœopaths (although numbers are increasing) experienced in treating people with HIV/AIDS, but these may usually be approached by contacting the local homœopathic association (details available from any good reference library).

United Kingdom
London Lighthouse
111-117 Lancaster Road,
London W11 1QT
Tel: 0171 792 1200
*Europe's largest centre for
people with HIV/AIDS. Offers
a wide variety of services
including a range of holistic
therapies.*

Terrence Higgins Trust
52 Grays Inn Road, London
WC1X 8JU
Tel: 0171 242 1010 (Helpline)
0171 404 2381 (Legal Line)
*Offers general advice on all
aspects of HIV/AIDS*

France
AIDES-Fédération
247 rue de Belleville,
75019 Paris
Tel: 1 44 52 00 00

Ireland
Body Positive
Dame House
24-26 Dame Street
Dublin 2
Tel: 1 671 24 04

USA
GMHC (Gay Men's Health
Crisis)
129 West 20th Street
New York
NY 10011
Tel: 212 807 66 64
Helpline: 212 807 66 55

Germany
Berliner AIDS-Hilfe
Meinekestraße 12
10719 Berlin
Tel: 30 883 30 17
Helpline: 30 194 11

Italy
ANLAIDS
Via Barberini 3
00187 Roma
Tel: 6 482 09 99
Helpline: 6 44 23 47 83

Netherlands
AIDS infolijn (AIDS helpline)
Polderweg 92
1093 KP Amsterdam
Tel: 06 022 22 20

Spain
FASE
Juan Montalvo 6
28040 Madrid
Tel: 1 536 15 00
Helpline: 900 11 10 00

New Zealand
New Zealand AIDS
Foundation, PO Box 6663
Wellesley Street
Auckland
Tel: 9 303 31 24
Helpline: 9 378 98 06

Australia
ACON (AIDS Council of New
South Wales)
PO Box 350
Darlinghurst
NSW 2010
Tel: 2 206 20 00

Aconite 20, 41, 45
Adrenal Cortex 111
Agnus Castus 59
Aids Nosode 60
Alfalfa 74, 78, 111
Aloe Vera 57
Ambra Grisea 41, 64, 74
Anacardium 46, 87, 88, 98
Anthracinum 64
A.C.T. Hormone 28, 111
Argentum Nitricum 41, 45
Arnica 5, 6, 20
Arsenicum 41, 45, 46, 64, 65, 66, 70, 72, 74, 83, 87, 89, 94
Aurum 17, 41, 46, 69, 88
Avena sativa 111
AZT 6, 7
Baryta Carbonica 76
Berberine containing herbs 57
Berberis Aquifolium 57
Berberis Vulgaris, 57
Bifidobacteria 57
Billy Goat Plum 27
Borax 56
Bromium 46, 69
Bryonia 111
Calcarea Arsenicosum 26, 45, 65, 70, 72
Calcarea Bromatum 46, 67
Calcarea Carbonica 17, 45, 66, 67, 76, 82
Calcarea Phosphorica 71, 98
Calcarea Sulphurica 45, 71
Calendula 5, 6
Candida Albicans 30, 54
Caprylic acid 57
Caprystatin 57
Carbo Vegetabilis 55, 65, 72, 73, 79, 83
Carbon Dioxide 84
Carcinosin 5, 6, 7, 17, 18, 28, 30, 31, 34, 41, 45, 46, 64, 69, 72, 80, 98
Carduus Marianus 26, 111

Caulophyllum 26
Causticum 34
Chelidonium 26, 54, 111
China 59, 72, 73, 85, 111
China Arsenicosum 65
China Boliviana 73
Cocculus 64
Coffea 23, 74
Cortisone 28, 55
Coxsackie Virus 30
Crotalus Horridus 34
Cryptococci 30
Cryptosporidium 30
Cundurango 77
Cytomegalovirus 30
Dys. Co 45
Echinacea 5, 6, 64, 75
Epstein-Barr virus 30
Erythromycin 55
Folliculinum 55
Fraxinus Americanus 26
Fucus Vesiculosus 26, 111
Gallium Apyrene 77
Garlic 58
Gorse 27
Granite 88
Graphites 71
Herpes Virus 30
Hydrastis 26, 57, 73, 76, 77, 111
Hypercal 21
Hypericum 5
Hypothalamus 28
Ignatia 41, 45, 64, 74, 87, 94, 98
Iodum 26, 111
Kali Bichromicum 81
Kali Muriaticum, 56
Lac Caninum 89
Lachesis 81
Lactobacillus Acidophilus 57
Lecithin 78
Leprominium 30, 78
Lilium Tigrinum 26

Liver 28, 111
Lycopodium 54, 55, 59, 73, 79
Macrocarpa 28
Malandrinum 5, 6
Malaria 30
Mandragora 55
Medorrhinum 28, 30, 69, 73, 79, 82, 87, 111
Medorrhinum Americana 80
Mercurius 18, 20, 24, 30, 32, 46, 64, 67, 69, 80, 81, 82, 95
Mercurius Corrosivus 32, 80, 83
Mercurius Iodatus Flavus 81
Mercurius Iodatus Ruber 81
Muriatic Acid 82
Mycobacteria 30
Mycopryl 56
Natrum Muriaticum 18, 69, 82, 88, 89, 94
Natrum Phosphoricum 56, 84
Natrum Sulphuricum 82
Nitricum Acidum 6, 83, 88
Nitrogen 84
Nux Vomica 26, 46, 72, 87, 88, 110, 111
Nystatin 55, 57
Oestrogen 55
Okoubaka 110
Oleic acid 58
Opium 20, 111
Pancreas 28
Penicillin 55
Phosphoric Acid 41, 46, 59, 85
Phosphorus 6, 7, 31, 34, 45, 67, 72, 84, 88
Picric Acid 59
Pituitary 28
Pneumocystis Carinii 30
Proteus 45, 46, 87
Pulsatilla 19, 26, 98, 110
Pyrogen 5, 6, 64, 88
Quercus Glandium 26
Radium Bromide 88
Rhus Toxicodendron 88
Rock Rose 27

Selenium 59
Self-Heal 27
Sepia 26, 55
Septrin 18
Serotonin 55
Silica 34
Spinifex 28
Spruce 27
Stannum 89
Staphylococci 31
Staphysagria 6, 18, 32, 87, 98
Stramonium 18, 20, 23, 45
Streptococci 30
Sulphur 18, 19, 23, 24, 73, 110
SVA 90
Sweet Chestnut 27
Syphilinum 20, 23, 28, 31, 41, 45, 46, 69, 73, 81, 89, 90, 94
Taheebo 57
Tarentula Cub 64
Tea Tree Oil 57
Thalamus 28
Thuja 25, 28, 30, 32, 46, 69, 73, 80, 82, 87, 91
Thymus Gland 31, 91, 99, 111
Thyreostimuline 55
Thyroidinum 26, 111
Toxoplasma Gondii 30
Tuberculinum 6, 7, 18, 23, 28, 31, 71, 73, 80, 85, 94
Tuberculinum Aviare 95
Tuberculinum. 94
Typhoidinum 30, 95
Urinum Humanum 28
Vanadium Mettallicum 96
Veratrum Album 6, 7
Vitamin B Complex 56
Vitamin C 56
Walnut 27
Wild Rose 27
X-ray 99

Abdominal distension 67
Abscesses 70, 74, 81
Absent menses 25
Acne 66
Acute conditions 12
Acyclovir 4, 100, 104
Adrenal cortex 102
Aetiologies 24
Aids 94
Alan Jones 46, 48, 88
Alcoholism 74
Allen 91
Aloe vera 53
Amphotericin 98
Amyl nitrate 77
Anaemia 72, 89, 96
Anger and frustration 42
Anorexia 89
Antibacterial 107
Antibiotics 31, 48, 66, 68, 75, 78, 101
Antidepressants 107
Antiepileptics 107
Antimalarial 106
Antiprotozoal 106
Anxiety 60
Arthritis 74
Australian bush 26
Auto-isopathy and Sarcodes 27
Azidothymidine 60
AZT 4, 60, 96, 104
Bach 26
Bailey 26
Barbara brennan 84
Bed sores 81
Benetton 1
Berberine containing herbs 53
Berberis aquifolium 53
Berberis vulgaris, 53
Bifidobacteria 53
Bill McGurk 55
Bleeding 74
Bleeding gums 75
Blindness 89

Blood 27
Boericke 91
Boils 59, 70
Bowel cancer 4
Bowel flora 48
Brain disease 64
Bronchitis 88
Bronchoconstriction 95
Bulimia 89
Californian 26
Cancer 71, 83
Candidiasis 76, 96, 102, 106
Caprylic acid 53
Caprystatin 52
Carbuncles 59, 70
Cerebral lymphoma 97
Chemo-therapy 91, 102
Chloroquin 100
Chronic constipation 71
Chronic diarrhoea 68
Chronic fatigue 91
Chronic grief 71
Chronic malaria 65
Clindamycin 104
Co-trimoxazole 107
Codeine phosphate 17, 105
Colin Griffiths 86
Combinations 25
Confusion 69
Conjunctivitis 75
Constitutional prescribing 24
Convalescence 66, 72
Convalescence. 67
Convulsions 97
Cortisone 17, 101
Cough 95
Cryptococcal meningitis 106
Cryptococcus neoformans 98
Cryptosporidium. 96
Cystitis 51
Cytomegalovirus 92, 95, 97, 106
Dapsone 105
DDC 105

DDI 100, 105
Dementia 98
Depression 41, 54, 98
DF 118 5, 105
Diarrhœa 22, 94, 96,105
Didanosine 105
Disorientation 69
Dr G Orth 46
Dr George F. Solomon 40
Dr Orion Truss 48
Dr. Prakash Vakil 72
Dr. Stephen Caiazza 83
Drainage 25
Drugs 100
Eclectic 14
Edward Bach 35
Edwin Steinbrecher xi
Eizayaga 15
Emaciation 89
Emotional trauma 69
Encephalitis 97
Endocrine system 102
Enlarged lymph glands 97
Family heredity 47
Fatigue 94
Fear and anxiety 41
Fear of death 65
Fevers 94
Fish fingers 78
Fissures 6, 77
Fistulas 77
Flatulence 67
Flower essences 12, 26
Fluconazole 4, 106
Folliculitis 96
Fungal infections 106
Ganciclovir 106
Garlic 53
Gastrocoat 4
Gonorrhœa 9, 47, 54, 74, 78
Grief 69, 87
Guilt 42
Gum disease 96
Haematuria 30
Haemophiliac 29

Haemorrhage 29
Hairy leukoplakia 96
Harris Coulter 83
Heart disease 74
Heartburn 78
Hemiplegia 97
Herpes 82, 92, 94
Herpes zoster 84
Herpes simplex 96
Human immunodeficiency virus 92
Human papilloma virus 96
Hydrastis 53
Immujem-SVA-30 83
Imodium 4
Impotence 54
Influenza 82
Insomnia 72
James Compton Burnett 10
Jan Scholten 63, 70, 89
John Diamond 85
Julie Williams 92
Kaposi's sarcoma 27, 73, 77, 83, 95, 97
Kentian 14
Ketoconazole 96, 106
Kidney drainage 25
Kidneys 65
Korsakoff 50
Lactobacilli 48
Lactobacillus acidophilus 51, 53
Lactulose 5
Layers 15
Leprosy 73, 105
Leucopenia 95
Liver 20, 50, 73, 102
Liver drainage 25
Lm potency 20
Low potency support 25
Lymphadenopathy 96
Lymphocytes 92
Lymphomas 97
MAI 79
Malaria 105
Manic depression 74

Marc Blausten 55
Miasms 27
Migraines 78
Mollusci 77
Molluscum contagiosum 96
Moriz Kaposi 84
Morphine 101, 103
Mouth ulcers 75
Multiple nosodes 29
Murdo Macdonald-Bayne 32
Mycobacterium avium
intracellulare 96
Mycopryl 52
Naproxen 5
Nausea 6, 50, 78
Nervous exhaustion 80
Neuro-retinitis 89
Night sweats 22, 68, 88, 94
Non Hodgkin's lymphoma 97
Nosodes 27
NSU 74
Nystatin 52
Obsessive disorders 42
Oleic acid 53
Ophthalmia 75
Opportunistic infections 100
Oral hairy leukoplakia 79
Oral thrush 51
Organ remedies 25
Pancreas 65
PCP 72, 78, 79, 87, 88, 95, 101,
105, 106
Penicillin 83
Pentamidine 4, 95, 106
Personal medical history 47
PGL - persistent generalised
Lymphadenopathy 94
Phatak 76
Phenytoin 107
Pneumocystis carinii pneumonia
95
Pneumonia 4, 79, 98
Post nasal catarrh 75
Post-nasal drip 94

Premature old age 54
Prescribing 10
Profound weakness 67
Prostate 54
Psoriasis 66, 96
Psychological issues 38
Pyremethamine 106, 107
Radiation 81
Radio-therapy 102
Radionics 55
Rajan Sankaran 65, 88
Raymond Charles Barker 8
Recreational drug abuse 47
Rectal herpes 4, 6, 77
Rectal ulcer 77
Respiratory disorders 95
Retinitis 97
Retroviruses 92
Rheumatism 74
Rifanal 107
Rocking 30
Samuel Hahnemann 15, 108
Scott J. Gregory 83
Seborrheic dermatitis 94, 96
Septicaemia 59, 70
Septrin 17, 78, 95, 101, 105,
107
Sexual abuse 55
Sexual excess 54
Shereen Joshua 55
Shingles 4
Shock 41, 65
Sinus 75
Skin conditions 96
Spiritual pathology 27
Steroids 102, 103
Stomach ulcers 75
Sulphadiazine 106, 107
Syphilis 47, 74, 83
Systemic candidiasis 48
Taheebo 53
Tea tree oil 53
The Healing Power Within 43
Thrush 96

Thymus gland 91
Thyroid 102
Thyroid support 25
Tinea (ringworm) 96
Tonsillitis 82, 88
Toxicity 81
Toxoplasmosis 97, 106, 107
Tuberculosis 87, 96, 105
Ulceration 81
Ulcers 74, 77, 81, 91, 96
Urine therapy 27
Vaccination 47, 70, 84, 102
Vaginal herpes 75
Vaginitis 51
Varicella zoster 96
Venereal diseases 47, 74
Vomiting 6, 68
Warts 96
Wasting 72, 88, 96
Weight loss 94
X rays 91
Zalcitabine 105
Zidovudine 60, 104
Zidovudine (AZT) 60, 95, 100,104

1 *The Inner Guide Meditation,* Edwin C. Steinbrecher.

2 Patient groups in USA: Homosexual/bisexual men: 65.1%; Intravenous drug abusers: 16.3%; Other: 18.6%. Source: *AIDS*, Williams, Mindel, Weller.

3 *The Astrologer's Handbook,* Francis Sakoian and Louis S. Acker.

4 *Treat Yourself to Life,* Raymond Charles Barker.

5 *The Best of Burnett*, James Compton Burnett,

6 Paragraph 274b of *The Organon* (suppressed from 5th edition) as quoted in *A Homœopathic Love Story* by Rima Handley.

7 *Treatise On Homœopathic Medicine,* F. Eizayaga.

8 An extract from this chapter together with a discussion on this way of prescribing may be found in *The Homœopath* no:63 1996.from The Society of Homœopaths, 2 Artizan Road, Northampton, England.

9 *Spiritual and Mental Healing,* Murdo MacDonald-Bayne.

10 *Medical Discoveries of Edward Bach*, Nora Weeks.

11 *What Doctors Don't Tell You* , edited by Lynn McTaggart, Vol ume 1 , no.7

12 *The ABC of AIDS*, 3rd Edition, Michael W. Adler.

13 Thanks to Robert Davidson for this analogy.

14 The Remedy Machine can be obtained from McGurk Electrical Services, 172 Leach Green Lane, Rednal, Birmingham, B45 8EH, England Tel: 0121-453 9898

15 Jan Scholten, *Homœopathy and Minerals*,

16 Rajan Sankaran, *The Substance of Homœopathy.*

17 Rajan Sankaran, *The Spirit of Homœopathy*

18 Jan Scholten, *Homœopathy and Minerals*,

19 Roger van Zandvoort, *The Complete Repertory*,

20 Robin Murphy, *Repertory*

21 *The Emerging Picture Of Leprominium: The Leprosy Nosode*, Dr. P. Vakil, IFH Professional Case Conference.1991 .

22 Helios Homœopathic Pharmacy, 97 Camden Road, Tunbridge, Kent

23 Fully discussed in *Prometheus Unbound*, vol 2 no2 Spring 1996. Available half-yearly from Jill Wright, The Rectory, Claremont Crescent, Crayford DA1 4RJ

24 *Materia Medica*, Phatak S

25 *Psychoimmunity and the Healing Process* by Jason Serinus (editor) 3rd Edition

26 Available from LAVO-VANDA-nv, TOEVLUCHTWEG 11 B8620, Nieupoort, Belgium.

27 *A Holistic Protocol for the Immune System* 6th Edition by Scott J. Gregory.

28 *Syphilis and AIDS*, Harris Coulter

29 *What the Doctors don`t tell you*

30 *Light Emerging*, Barbara Brennan

31 *Life Energy*, John Diamond

32 *Prometheus Unbound*, vol. 2 no.1 Autumn 1995.

33 *Substance of Homœopathy*, p.57.Rajan Sankaran

34 *Homœopathy and Minerals*, Jan Scholten

35 *Materia Medica*, Boericke

36 *Materia Medica of the Nosodes with X ray Provings*, Allen H C

37 *Repertory,* Robin Murphy

38 A description of this remedy is given in *Prometheus Unbound* vol. 1 no. 1, June 1994.

39 *Medicines-The Comprehensive Guide*, 3rd Edition, Dr Ian Morton and Dr Judith Hall.

40 *Organon of Medicine*, 6th Edition, Samuel Hahnemann.